FOOD FOR SPORT

A HANDBOOK OF SPORTS NUTRITION

Peter Berry Ottaway BSc CBiol MIBiol FIFST FRSH

Kevin Hargin BSc PhD AIFST

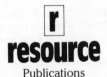

resource
Publications

43–45 Hobson Street
Cambridge CB1 1NL

First published 1985 by Resource Publications Basic Skills Unit Ltd

British Library Cataloguing in Publication Data

Ottaway, Peter Berry
    Food for sport: a handbook of sports nutrition.
    1. Athletes — Nutrition
    I. Title   II. Hargin, Kevin
    641.1'024796   TX361.A8

   ISBN 0 948784 00 8

Photoset by Hobson Street Studio Limited, 44a Hobson Street, Cambridge CB1 1NL

Printed by The Burlington Press, Foxton, Cambridge

Contents

List of tables

List of illustrations

Acknowledgements

The authors wish to thank the following for their generous assistance and support in the preparation of the book:

Dr Derek Shrimpton
Dr James Scala
Dr Steve Wootton
for their help and advice

Shaklee Corporation
for the use of the data in chapter 15

Andrea Berry Ottaway
for patiently preparing and typing the manuscript

The many sportsmen and women who have generously helped us and other researchers in developing the approaches outlined in this book.

Peter Berry Ottaway
Kevin Hargin
December 1985

How to use *Food for sport*

Food for sport is a highly condensed yet readable collation of current knowledge about nutrition and sport. Our recommendation is that you should read *all* of it, except possibly the three chapters (10–12) which deal with specialised subjects. If you are familiar with nutritional principles, there are probably things in the book that are new to you. If you are not, use it as an introduction in the confident knowledge that you are in touch with the 'state of the art'.

Overview

1   *Food and sport*
Sets the scene.

2 and 3   *Nutrients and digestion*
An overview of current knowledge. Skim through to refresh or update yourself; read carefully if you are new to it.

4 and 5   *Energy*
Incorporates a great deal of current thinking on energy metabolism. Essential for all readers.

6 and 7   *Vitamins and minerals*
Removes many misconceptions about these, and summarises the current state of knowledge. Essential for all readers.

8 and 9   *Fluid balances and body weight*
Crucial material for safety, especially in endurance sports.

10 to 12   *Special interests*
Describes requirements for teenagers and diabetic athletes, and special techniques such as carbohydrate loading.

13 to 15   *Theory into practice*
Puts it all together in a practical way. Includes menu planning, meal selection and a case study of the American Ski Team.

There is also a glossary, appendices, a complete reference section for those who wish to check the original research or go further into the subject, and an index.

This book

The aim of this book is to give an outline of the scientific background to the principles of sports nutrition and to give sound advice on the development of a sports diet. Chapters 2 and 3 give a brief résumé of the classifications and the roles of the various nutrients in food and the processes by which these nutrients are digested and absorbed into the body. It is important to have this appreciation of the basic principles of nutrition because they provide the foundation on which the more specialised ideas of sports nutrition are built. Of necessity in a small handbook of this type some of the nutritional background has had to be dealt with more superficially than the authors would have liked, and some aspects, not totally relevant to the understanding of the rest of the text, have had to be omitted. If you require more detailed information look at the references and textbooks listed at the end of the book.

In common with current scientific thinking, the book does not attempt to define a range of sports-specific diets. The idea of having a special diet for each sport or group of allied sports has been very popular for some time, and has in the main been based on misguided perception of protein requirements.

There is substantial scientific evidence that diet can have a significant effect on endurance capacity, and inherently performance, and adherence to a well-designed diet should be an important part of any sports training programme. Like any other training technique benefits are unlikely to be instantaneous but will accrue over time.

All athletes will benefit by keeping to the general principles outlined in the book.

1 Food and sport

We are now living in an era when sport, both professional and amateur, has entered the truly international arena and an increasing number of sportsmen and women are taking part in competitions where titles and records are won or lost on the smallest fractions of a second or centimetre.

In their constant striving for perfection in their chosen sport, athletes are experimenting with all the variables that can affect performance including footwear, clothing and training techniques. It is therefore surprising to find in many cases that only scant attention has been paid to diet. One of the reasons for this neglect is probably that until recently there has been very little public awareness of the impact of diet on health, and virtually no sound information on the effect of diet on performance.

Although food-gathering is mankind's oldest occupation, the science of nutrition has tended to be the poor relation of the biological and medical sciences. Nutritional training in schools has either been made a small part of domestic science and home economics courses or neglected altogether. British universities only began to offer full-time first degree courses in nutrition in the 1960s, and nutrition still represents only an extremely small portion of the medical syllabus. As a consequence most people have had little training in this important subject.

The emergence of official reports in the 1980s linking nutritional habits to a number of diseases has created recent public interest in the necessity, among other things, to increase the fibre and reduce the fat content of the diet. The debate on the two principal reports, the Health Education Council paper, *Proposals for nutritional guidelines for health education in Britain* (National Advisory Committee on Nutritional Education – NACNE) issued in 1983, and the *Report on diet and cardiovascular disease,* known as the COMA report (Committee on Medical Aspects of Food), issued in 1984, proved a bonus for the media and has resulted in an avalanche of television and radio programmes, books and articles. This sudden onslaught of information has left people confused. For the previous 20 to 30 years the emphasis had been on reduction of carbohydrates in the diet and many companies prospered from selling starch-reduced breads and biscuits. Advice in slimming publications was to avoid sugar and starches, and a whole generation has grown up with the idea that starch is fattening. In addition protein was seen as a very important component of the diet.

It may come as a shock to today's athletes to be told to considerably increase the starch component of their diets, to reduce the fat, and to ease off on the protein.

Relatively recent research on the way energy is stored and used by the body has led to the development of new concepts in sports nutrition, and emphasis is now placed on the intake of starch-based products to build up energy reserves for endurance sports. The traditional high intake of proteins, particularly by those participating in sports requiring strength, is being discouraged and a reduction in the fat content of the diet is recommended for all athletes. In addition more emphasis is now being placed on the intake of water and the water balance within the body.

2 The role of nutrients in food

We eat to live. We eat to grow, reproduce and to lead a full healthy life. Human beings have a tremendous advantage over all other animals in that we have exploited a vast range of food sources and are able to manipulate food to gratify our sight, taste and smell; quite apart from satisfying the primary instinct of hunger. There has been a tendency in the developed countries to produce foods to sensory rather than nutritional criteria, but it is the nutritional aspect of the food that keeps us alive.

To have a healthy existence we must obtain over 40 important nutrients from our food, and it is essential that we obtain these regularly and in the right amounts.

If we want to develop our bodies to a high level of physical fitness and performance, we need a basic understanding of nutritional requirements and the effect various nutrients can have on the body.

To do this, start thinking of food in terms of its nutrient composition and balance food sources during the day to give the best chance of taking in the required nutrients. Start to see food not only in terms of its form, texture and taste, but also as a contributor of energy, protein, vitamins and minerals, together with 'bulk' or dietary fibre.

The composition of food

Food serves a number of purposes in the body and to do this it must contain substances that function in one or more of three ways:

provide fuel to the body in the form of energy

provide material for the building or maintenance of body tissues

supply substances that act to regulate the wide range of body processes.

Food consists of seven basic categories of nutrients. These are classified by their function in the body and not by chemical composition, and are carbohydrates, fats, proteins, vitamins, minerals, fibre and water (fig 1). The first three groups – carbohydrates, fats and protein – are also known as the 'energy nutrients' since, except for alcohol, these are the only compounds from which the body can derive energy for work and heat.

Carbohydrates

These are an important source of energy for the body's cells and organs. Within this class fall the sugars and starches, and all the compounds are characterised by being made up of the elements carbon, hydrogren and oxygen, with the hydrogen and oxygen almost always present in the two-to-one ratio found in water. This gave rise to the name carbo- (carbon) hydrate (water). The majority of carbohydrates are derived from plants where they are formed from carbon dioxide, water and energy from the sun by a process known as photosynthesis. The simplest carbohydrates are the simple sugars such as glucose or fructose. The cane or beet sugar we commonly use is formed by combining two simple sugars, and starches are made of a number of simple sugars linked together to form long chains (fig 2).

Whilst carbohydrates can be found with a variety of different chain lengths, they are broken down by the body's digestive system to simple sugars such as glucose before being absorbed into the body.

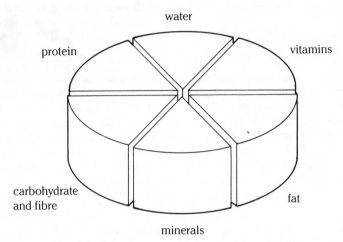

Fig 1 *The essential nutrients in foods*

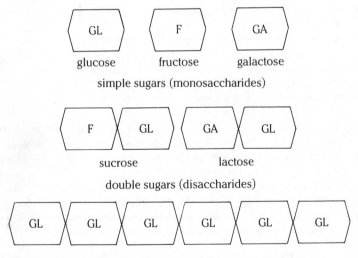

Fig 2 *Diagrammatic representation of the hexose carbohydrates showing the formation of monosaccharides, disaccharides and polysaccharides*

3

The glucose is absorbed through the intestines into the blood where it is maintained at a steady concentration. It may then either be transported to the body cells to be used directly for energy or converted to glycogen and stored in the liver and muscles as an energy reserve or, if the body has taken in sufficient carbohydrate to meet immediate energy demands, the surplus can be converted to triglycerides and stored as adipose tissue (body fat).

At the cellular level, glucose is oxidised to give energy to the equation:

$$\text{glucose} + \text{oxygen} \rightarrow \text{energy} + \text{carbon dioxide} + \text{water}$$

More about this energy release will be covered in the next chapter.

In addition to the groups of carbohydrates which contribute energy, there are a number of other compounds which come under the general classification of carbohydrate. These include the complex polysaccharides which are found in plant matter; examples of these are cellulose, hemicellulose and a variety of plant gums and mucilages. Most of these compounds are not broken down in the human digestive system and pass through the gut to be excreted in faeces. The complex polysaccharides are the components of dietary fibre (see page 12).

Fats

Fat is a much maligned and misunderstood nutrient. We are urged by the medical profession and nutritionists alike to cut down our fat intake, particularly animal fats and, as a result, fat has become regarded by most people as being unhealthy. However, it is important to realise that not only are certain fats essential but the amounts and proportions of different types of fat are also significant.

Like carbohydrates, fats are made up of carbon, oxygen and hydrogen, but the proportion of oxygen is much lower in fats than carbohydrates. Fats are a concentrated source of energy and can be stored in the body as an energy reserve.

True fats are made up of glycerol combined with either one, two or three fatty acids to give mono-, di-, and triglycerides respectively. The differences between one fat and another are largely the result of differences in the fatty acids.

The term lipid is often used interchangeably with fat but while all fats are lipids not all lipids are fats. In addition to fats lipids also include related substances such as waxes, cholesterol, lecithin and other phospholipids. These are chemically more complex than fats but contain at least one fatty acid or fatty acid derivative. Oils usually refer to lipids which are liquid at room temperature.

The physical properties of fats are determined by the differences in kinds and amounts of fatty acids present. Fatty acids have different melting points and levels of hydrogen saturation. Although most people have little interest in the complex structure of the fatty acid molecules, these structural differences have nutritional significance.

Polyunsaturated fats, in general, are from vegetable sources and are liquid at room temperature (exceptions to this are coconut and cashew nut oils which are highly saturated) whereas saturated fats are normally firm or solid at room temperature and can be found in such foods as butter, lard and other animal fats (table 1).

The double bond in the polyunsaturated molecule can be broken through a

Table 1 *Major sources of cholesterol, saturated and polyunsaturated fats in the diet*

Cholesterol	Saturated fat	Polyunsaturated fat
egg yolk*	lard	sunflower seed oil
organ meats such as heart, brain, liver, kidney and sweetbreads	suet	corn (maize) oil
	pork and bacon dripping	cotton seed oil
shellfish (oysters, prawns, shrimps, crab, lobster)	mutton	peanut oil
	butter	soya bean oil
dairy products including butter, cheese, cream, milk	hard margarine	safflower oil
baked foods prepared with egg yolk, butter, or whole milk	hydrogenated vegetable oils	certain soft margarines such as those produced with sunflower oil
	coconut oil	most nuts except coconut and cashew
	hard cheeses	
	cream	

* Egg yolks are a particularly rich source of cholesterol in our diets.

chemical process called hydrogenation, which converts oils to a solid or semisolid form by increasing the amount of hydrogen saturation. Unsaturated fats are less stable than the saturated variety and the double bond linkages will react with atmospheric oxygen (ie oxidise) to make the fat rancid.

There are many fatty acids, but the two most important are linoleic acid and linolenic acid. These are called the 'essential fatty acids' because people need them in regular small quantities (1 to 2 per cent of total energy intake) to maintain normal health.

Another fatty acid which has gained prominence recently is eicosapentaenoic acid, more commonly called EPA. There is growing evidence to suggest that EPA alters blood platelet behaviour and bleeding time and may therefore reduce the possibility of intravascular thrombosis. Detailed research into the effects of EPA on different population groups has not yet been completed, and much of the evidence relating to EPA's beneficial effects has come from the observation that Greenland Eskimos and some Japanese coastal communities who have a diet rich in oily fish (which is a good source of EPA) also have a low incidence of coronary heart disease.

Fats are of value in our diet for a number of reasons. The most important being

as a source of essential fatty acids (this is the only *essential* use of fat in the diet; the other functions are desirable but not essential)

as a concentrated energy source

as carriers for the fat-soluble vitamins to aid their absorption

for satiety value, to give a feeling of fullness to the meal and suppress feelings of hunger

to improve the flavour of foods and to make them more appetising.

Studies on the incidence of disease in population groups (epidemiological studies) have provided evidence which links a high intake of saturated fat with coronary heart disease. The balance of current opinion is that the whole population should reduce saturated fat in the diet and increase the polyunsaturated fat component. In food terms this means reducing the intake of animal-derived fats such as meat fat, butter and lard, and increasing the consumption of vegetable oils (table 1). Many other factors are of course involved in the risk of heart disease. These include family history, obesity, smoking, stress, hypertension and lack of exercise.

Some lipids, principally cholesterol, have also been implicated in heart disease. It is widely believed that there is a relationship between high-serum cholesterol and risk of heart disease. Research also indicates that an increased intake of polyunsaturated fats coupled with a lower consumption of saturated fats can be helpful in reducing serum cholesterol.

The body does of course manufacture its own cholesterol which is used for example in the formation of certain hormones and bile acids, and in normal circumstances this production will be balanced against dietary intakes.

Another important group within the general term lipid is the phospholipids which incorporate a phosphorus-containing compound in place of the third fatty acid found in triglycerides.

The best known in this group is lecithin (phosphatidyl choline) which is found in all cell membranes and body tissues including the brain, liver and heart. Lecithin also has the role of an emulsifier in the body and aids absorption and transportation of fats and fat-soluble vitamins.

Commercially, the term lecithin refers to a mixture of phospholipids including phosphatidyl choline, cephalin (phosphatidyl ethanolamine) and phosphatidyl inositol. These are broken down in the body to their component parts of unsaturated fatty acids, choline, inositol and phosphorus.

Like all the nutrients, fat is neither good nor bad. Just as with protein and carbohydrate, the form and amount of fat must be considered in the light of variable individual factors that determine nutritional requirements.

Protein

Protein was one of the first nutrients to be discovered. It was recognised in the first half of the nineteenth century not only as a source of energy but also as an important nutrient. In fact, the name protein is derived from the Greek meaning 'to come first'.

All living matter, both plant and animal, discovered to date contains protein as it forms a vital part of every cell. Proteins are important in the structural and functional characteristics of all living tissues, and protein, in a myriad of forms, makes up more than half of all the organic matter in the human body.

The body's need for protein is never-ending. The tissues need a supply to stay healthy, and protein is also part of all the enzymes and some of the hormones that control digestion, growth, and the release of energy from food.

Proteins are composed of larger and more complex molecules than those of either fats or carbohydrates and are the only class of 'energy nutrients', with a few minor exceptions such as inositol among the lipids, that contain nitrogen in addition to carbon, hydrogen and oxygen. Most also contain sulphur and many contain phosphorus, iron or other minerals. Plants can synthesise proteins from simple inorganic compounds, but animals cannot synthesise all the components of protein and must get their protein from eating plants or from eating animals which have lived on plants.

The protein obtained from food cannot function in the body until it is broken down into its component parts, the amino acids. Some 22 different amino acids are fairly commonly present in proteins that occur in nature. Twenty of these are needed for the body's numerous protein combinations. Of this total, the body can form eleven which

Table 2   *Amino acids*

Essential amino acids	*Non-essential amino acids*
isoleucine	alanine
leucine	arginine
lysine	asparagine
methionine	aspartic acid
phenylalanine	cysteine
threonine	cystine
tryptophan	glutamic acid
valine	glutamine
histidine*	glycine
	hydroxyproline
	proline
	serine
	tyrosine

* Histidine is required for infants, but it has not been fully established that it is essential for adults.

are known as the 'non-essential' amino acids. Of the remaining nine, eight have to be obtained preformed in the diet and are known as 'essential amino acids'. The ninth, histidine, has been found to be essential for infants but it has not been fully established that it is essential for adults. Nonetheless, it is normally regarded as an essential amino acid (table 2).

It is important that all 'essential' amino acids are present in the food supply and also that they are present in the right proportions. It is only when all the 'essential' amino acids are present in required amounts that the body can build tissue protein and carry out its functions (fig 3).

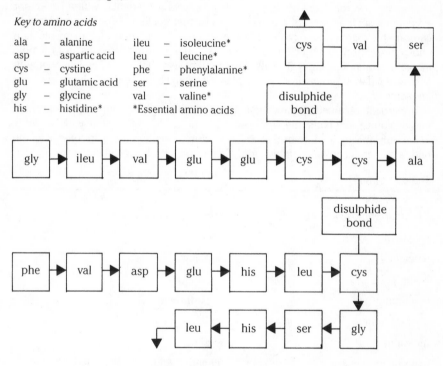

Key to amino acids

ala	–	alanine	ileu	–	isoleucine*
asp	–	aspartic acid	leu	–	leucine*
cys	–	cystine	phe	–	phenylalanine*
glu	–	glutamic acid	ser	–	serine
gly	–	glycine	val	–	valine*
his	–	histidine*			*Essential amino acids

(Adapted from Taylor 1964)

Fig 3   *Diagrammatic representation of part of the amino acid sequence in a molecule of protein (beef insulin)*

Over the years there has been much research and discussion on the relative quality of protein from different sources. As a number of plant proteins only contain small amounts of amino acids essential to humans and many other mammals, they were not considered to be complete proteins. A number of scientific methods of measuring protein quality were developed and most were based on animal feeding trials. In these trials either casein (milk protein) or egg protein were the standard against which other proteins were judged (table 3).

Table 3   *Relative protein nutritive values*

Protein source	Average assay value
casein (milk protein)	100
lactalbumins (milk protein)	99
egg white	115
textured soya protein	82
soya isolate unfortified with additional amino acids	71
peanut flour	67
wheat gluten	34

Nutritive values of various protein sources related to casein (casein = 100). Based on rat assay techniques.   (Adapted from Bodwell 1979)

Although these trials, which were mainly conducted on rats, show very significant differences in the quality of vegetable proteins when compared with animal proteins, the implications are now not considered to be so important for humans on a diet containing protein from a variety of sources.

Vitamins

Up to the beginning of this century it was thought that a diet which supplied protein, carbohydrates, fats, some minerals and water in suitable amounts was all that was necessary for normal nutrition. But in 1912 F G Hopkins published a paper giving results of experiments which suggested that there were other substances in addition to those already known which were essential to growth and life. He called these 'accessory growth factors'.

Subsequent research has identified 13 compounds which have now been called vitamins. These are organic compounds other than any of the amino acids, fatty acids or carbohydrates that need to be present in small amounts in the diet for maintaining health, growth and reproduction.

Unlike the nutrients we have already discussed, vitamins do not serve a structural or storage function or contribute energy to the body. They have a catalytic function, controlling the various metabolic processes in the body. Vitamins are compounds that help to trigger biochemical reactions in the body so that food can be converted into substances that can be used by the cells of the body tissues.

The 13 vitamins that have been discovered are all chemically distinct. Each plays a particular role or number of roles in maintaining the body processes, and no one vitamin is able to do the work of another. The lack of any one of the vitamins in the diet will lead to ill health and eventually to a deficiency disease.

9

Vitamins can be classified into two groups: fat-soluble and water-soluble. The first group contains vitamins A, D, E and K. The eight B-complex vitamins and vitamin C form the water-soluble group (table 4).

Table 4 *Vitamins*

Fat-soluble

vitamin A (retinol and axerophthol)

vitamin D (ergocalciferol and cholecalciferol)

vitamin E (tocopherol)

vitamin K (phytonadione and phytomenadione)

Water-soluble

vitamin B_1 (thiamin)

vitamin B_2 (riboflavin)

vitamin B_6 (pyridoxine)

vitamin B_{12} (cyanocobalamin)

niacin (nicotinic acid and nicotinamide)

pantothenic acid

biotin

folic acid

vitamin C (ascorbic acid)

The fat-soluble vitamins tend to be more stable to heat than the B-complex vitamins and vitamin C, and are less likely to be lost by cooking and processing food. As they are not soluble in water they are not excreted in the urine. But they can be stored to a considerable extent, mainly in the liver. The ability of the body to store fat-soluble vitamins, particulary A and D, can present a toxicity problem if large amounts are eaten continuously.

The water-soluble vitamins are not stored in appreciable amounts and any excess is excreted in the urine.

Many vitamins, particularly the fat-soluble ones, can occur in more than one closely related chemical form. As a consequence it was found in the early days of vitamin research that the different forms of the vitamin at a given amount did not produce exactly the same degree of biological effect in the body. Some method of biological standardisation was necessary, and the system of International Units (IU) was introduced. For example, within the vitamin E group of compounds, 1 International

Unit of viamin E is equivalent to

1 mg dl-α-tocopheryl acetate   *or*
0.909 mg dl-α-tocopherol   *or*
0.735 mg d-α-tocopheryl acetate *or*
0.671 mg d-α-tocopherol   *or*
1.75 mg d-β-tocopherol

Vitamins A, D and E can still have their values given in international units, although it is now becoming more acceptable to relate each form of the vitamin to a pure standard form. In the United Kingdom vitamin A is now quoted in microgrammes of pure retinol equivalent (retinol being the alcohol form of vitamin A).

Other vitamins are now measured in terms of milligrammes (mg) which are thousandths of a gramme, or microgrammes (mcg or μg) which represent millionths of a gramme.

Minerals

This large and important group of nutrients contains all the inorganic elements that our bodies need for both structural and biochemical purposes.

Minerals have three main functions:

as structural constituents of bones and teeth

as soluble salts which help to control the composition of body fluids; in this role they are called electrolytes

as essential adjuncts to many enzymes and hormones playing a part in numerous biochemical reactions.

Some minerals such as calcium, magnesium and phosphorus are present in the body in relatively large amounts and called macrominerals. The others which are needed in very small amounts are called trace minerals. The relative content of the various minerals in the body is given in table 5.

A mineral can have a number of functions within the body. For example, calcium is an essential component of the structure of bones and teeth. It is needed to trigger specific enzymatic reactions in the body, it plays a major role in maintaining muscle tone including the heart muscles, it is involved in nerve transmission, and it is required for normal clotting of the blood. It is also an important component of the body's electrolyte system.

The important macrominerals are calcium, phosphorus, sodium, potassium and magnesium. The element chlorine, although not strictly a mineral, is also required in substantial amounts.

The essential trace minerals are those needed in very small amounts (milligrammes or microgrammes per day) but nevertheless are essential for the proper maintenance of bodily functions. Trace minerals for which functions have been well established include iron, iodine, zinc, cobalt, copper, manganese, chromium, selenium, molybdenum and fluorine.

There are a number of minerals which are essential for other animal species, but

11

Table 5   *Major mineral content in the adult human body*

Element	Chemical symbol	Total ash (%)	Grammes per 70 kg body weight
calcium	Ca	39	1160
phosphorus	P	22	670
potassium	K	5	150
sulphur	S	4	112
chlorine	Cl	3	85
sodium	Na	2	63
magnesium	Mg	0.7	21
iron	Fe	0.15	4.5
zinc	Zn	0.007	2.0
iodine	I	0.0007	0.02

their function in humans is still unclear at our present state of knowledge. This group of minerals includes tin, nickel, silicon and vanadium. It is typical that a trace element that plays an essential role in one or more mammals will eventually prove to be essential in humans.

Dietary fibre

Dietary fibre is not strictly a nutrient as it is not absorbed into the body. However, fibre is derived from food sources and has been shown to play an important part in health and well-being.

Dietary fibre is the collective name given to a number of indigestible complex carbohydrates found in plant cell walls. Fibre is not broken down by the enzymes in the digestive system, and as it passes through the intestine it acts as a bulking agent and regulates the transit time of faeces.

Five groups of compounds are now thought to contribute dietary fibre. These are celluloses, hemicelluloses, lignins, pectins and gums. They are found in cereal products, vegetables, and fruits. All five components should be present in the diet to provide our fibre requirements.

It is only fairly recently that the importance of dietary fibre has been appreciated, and this was mainly due to the perception of Surgeon Captain T L Cleave of the Royal Navy and Dr Denis Burkitt. Captain Cleave demonstrated the beneficial effects of bran in reducing the incidence of constipation among the crew of a battleship during the second world war.

Dr Burkitt, who worked for 20 years as a surgeon in Africa, compared the incidence of bowel disease in an African population on a high cereal diet with Europeans on a typical western diet, and concluded that many problems of constipation, diverticular disease and bowel cancer in the Europeans could be attributed to their very much lower consumption of cereal products.

An examination of dietary habits in the United Kingdom over the past hundred years shows that our consumption of cereal products has more than halved since the beginning of this century.

Water

Water is second only to oxygen in importance to the body. A healthy adult can survive for weeks without food but only a few days without water. The average body water content in the general population is about 61 per cent of body weight. A loss of 6 per cent of the total body water is serious and a loss of 10 to 11 per cent is fatal.

Water is necessary for all the processes of digestion, absorption and nutrient transportation. Nutrients are dissolved in water to enable them to pass through the intestinal wall into the bloodstream for use throughout the body. Water also carries waste out of the body and helps to regulate body temperature.

3 Digestion

Putting food into the mouth initiates a series of chemical and physical processes which convert the animal and plant matter into nutrients the body needs.

Our normal meals are simply a combination of the basic nutrients: fats, proteins, carbohydrates, vitamins and minerals. Although a few foods are made up of only one nutrient, for example table sugar is pure carbohydrate, most foods are complex mixtures.

The process of digestion is to break down foods into simpler and simpler substances and prepare them for absorption into the body's tissues.

Digestion and absorption occur in a long tube called the alimentary tract which passes through the body and has openings to the exterior at each end (fig 4). The different surfaces and structures within this tract provide for the food to be broken down by the processes of digestion in the upper sections and then to be selectively absorbed in the lower sections.

The entrance to the alimentary tract is the mouth. Here our food is chewed and broken down into smaller particles and is also mixed with saliva. An enzyme in saliva begins breaking down the starches into simple sugars. This is the start of digestion whereby complex food molecules are gradually broken down into simpler units that can be absorbed by the body.

After the food has been chewed it is propelled to the back of the mouth by the tongue and then passes through the oesophagus by waves of contractions, known as peristalsis, to the stomach.

In the stomach, food is changed both physically and chemically by the gastric juices and the kneading contractions of muscles in the stomach walls. The stomach also contains hydrochloric acid which creates the proper acidity for the digestion of protein, activates the gastric enzyme protease and increases the solubility of certain minerals such as iron and calcium. Gastric secretions also contain a substance called mucin which protects the lining of the stomach from the hydrochloric acid.

Peristalsis continues to move food in a solution known as chyme through the alimentary tract. The upper part of the stomach is muscularly inactive and acts as a reservoir where food may remain for some time before it is gradually pushed toward the pylorus, the outlet of the stomach.

From time to time, the pylorus opens and a peristaltic wave flushes a portion of chyme into the first part of the small intestine called the duodenum. The rate at which the stomach empties is chiefly dependent upon the types of food we eat. Liquids leave the stomach relatively quickly. Concentrated foods and foods with high fibre content are retained longer. In general, carbohydrate foods leave the stomach first, followed by the proteins and then fats last of all.

The average time for the stomach to empty of an ordinary meal is about three hours. When the stomach is empty for a long period strong rhythmic contractions begin, giving the familiar hunger pangs. A meal that contains some fat, or fat and protein, can delay these hunger contractions, an important fact for dieters to know.

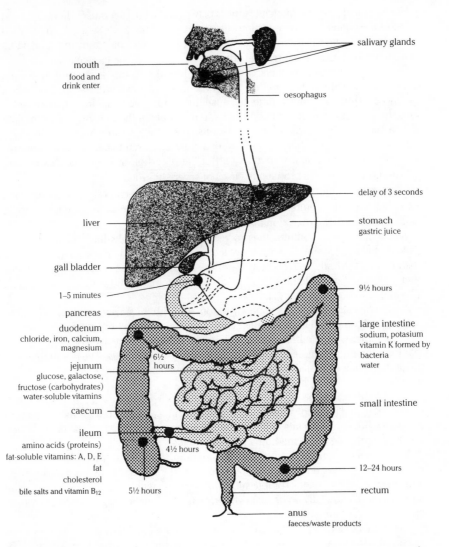

mouth
food and
drink enter

salivary glands

oesophagus

liver

delay of 3 seconds

stomach
gastric juice

gall bladder

1–5 minutes

9½ hours

pancreas

duodenum
chloride, iron, calcium,
magnesium

large intestine
sodium, potassium
vitamin K formed by
bacteria
water

6½
hours

jejunum
glucose, galactose,
fructose (carbohydrates)
water-soluble vitamins

caecum

small intestine

ileum
amino acids (proteins)
fat-soluble vitamins: A, D, E
fat
cholesterol
bile salts and vitamin B_{12}

4½ hours

12–24 hours

5½ hours

rectum

anus
faeces/waste products

Note: times indicate period taken for first part of meal to reach the various sections of the alimentary canal after leaving the mouth.

Fig 4   *Digestive tract showing nutrient absorption sites*

It is in the small intestine that most of the food is broken down into its constituent parts and absorbed into the body.

When the chyme passes into the duodenum, the action triggers the release of bile from the gall bladder and pancreatic juices from the pancreas.

Muscular action in the small intestine is of two kinds. Circular muscle fibres mix and squeeze the contents of the intestine against the intestinal walls so they can be acted upon by the digestive enzymes. Longitudinal fibres maintain the peristaltic movements that move the intestinal contents along toward the large intestine.

Transit time for the contents of the small intestine varies according to several factors. The amount of fibre in the food certainly plays a major role – the more fibre, the more rapid the transit time because the bulk gives the intestinal muscles something to move along. Irritating or toxic materials in the intestine can stimulate peristalsis so radically that diarrhoea results (the condition in which food residues pass through the intestine so rapidly that they are excreted in fluid condition). Normally, the fluid is reabsorbed as part of the digestion process. For this reason, dehydration is a serious problem in cases of severe diarrhoea.

Carbohydrate digestion begins in the mouth. By the time carbohydrate foods reach the small intestine, complex carbohydrates have already begun to resemble simple sugars because of the digestion that started with the saliva.

Intestinal enzymes continue the process until all the carbohydrates in the meal are broken down into simple sugars (glucose, galactose and fructose) that can be absorbed by the body. The carbohydrates are ready to be absorbed about 30 minutes after they enter the small intestine. The fats and proteins are much more complex and take longer to digest.

Protein digestion, which began in the stomach with the enzyme pepsin, and other enzymes, is completed in the small intestine. Enzymes which flow into the duodenum from the pancreas and others that come from the small intestine itself break the chains that form the protein molecules into the individual amino acids. These amino acids, the building blocks of all living cells, are then able to pass into the cells lining the small intestine.

Fat digestion, in the watery environment of the digestive tract, is the most complicated and time-consuming of all. The churning action in the stomach results in a coarse emulsion of the fats and the stomach also produces the enzyme lipase which breaks down some of the medium-chain fatty acids.

As this coarse emulsion enters the duodenum from the stomach it triggers the release of pancreatic enzymes that break down the fat molecules into three fatty acids and glycerol. As only water-soluble substances can penetrate the watery surface of the intestinal walls, the fatty acids must go through additional changes, assisted by bile, before they can be absorbed.

Bile is manufactured by the liver and stored in the gall bladder. When fatty food passes into the small intestine bile flows in and the salts in bile hold the fatty acids in a suspension. These are able to pass through the intestinal wall membranes.

The fatty acids are then formed into aggregates called chylomicrons. These consist of the fatty acids, phosphatidyl choline and lipoproteins. The chylomicrons are transported across the intestinal cells and are released into the intercellular spaces where they enter the lymphatic system.

What is left are the micronutrients and waste products. The micronutrients are absorbed directly into the blood.

The main part of the small intestine is called the jejunum and is covered with tiny finger-like projections called villi. The biggest are around 1 mm long (1/25th of an inch). Each tiny villus consists of cells porous enough to allow simple molecules to pass through. Inside each is a blood vessel that carries away glucose and amino acids. Food that brushes against the villi is digested by the enzymes and then absorbed. The vitamins in food are not broken down further by the digestive process. They are simply absorbed directly into the blood.

Much of the fluid in our food and drink as well as many minerals are not absorbed until they reach the large intestine, which also receives all indigestible remnants of the food.

Approximately 5 per cent or less of an average meal ends up as waste product which arrives in the large intestine as a spongy mass. Muscular action continues to push it through the last section of intestine known as the colon. The water is absorbed from it during its passage to the rectum. The remaining mass, now called faeces, causes pressure in the rectum which leads to defaecation.

You will probably appreciate that digestion is a complex process involving numerous biochemical reactions and taking many hours to accomplish. An awareness of the timescale is very important to people doing sports as the food has to be consumed a number of hours before the event for maximum benefit to be derived from the meal.

4 Energy and the energy nutrients

All living organisms require energy, which can be defined as the power to do work. Energy exists in a number of forms; for example heat, light, sound and electricity are familiar forms. Energy can also be stored in chemical forms such as in a car or torch battery.

The energy used by our bodies comes in the form of potential chemical energy stored in foods. This energy originates from the sun and is converted by green plants into the organic compounds now familiar to us as carbohydrates. Green plants synthesise organic compounds from water and carbon dioxide by photosynthesis, a process which uses energy absorbed from sunlight.

All our energy is obtained either directly or indirectly from plant sources. We get it directly by eating vegetables, fruits and cereal products, or indirectly from the consumption of animals which have obtained their energy from eating plants.

Measuring energy

The energy provided by foods is measured in kilocalories (kcal) or kiloJoules (kJ). A calorie is defined as the heat required to raise the temperature of 1 g of water through 1 degree centigrade. As this unit is relatively small, nutritionists quote the energy values of foods in kilocalories (1 kilocalorie = 1000 calories). Although calories are the most widely known unit of energy the Joule is the energy unit now generally accepted by scientists. The Joule is a unit of work (1 Joule = 10^7 ergs) and 1000 Joules make 1 kiloJoule. 1 kilocalorie is equivalent to 4.184 kiloJoules. The accepted conversion factors in the United Kingdom for converting weights of energy nutrients to energy are:

	Energy per gramme	
	kilocalories	kiloJoules
carbohydrates	3.75	16
fats	9.00	37
protein	4.00	17
alcohol	7.00	29

1 g of fat, therefore, contains over twice the energy found in a gramme of carbohydrate or protein.

Converting energy

The energy nutrients (carbohydrate, fat, protein and alcohol) are converted to energy by complex biochemical reactions known as 'Krebs cycle' to form a compound: adenosine triphosphate (ATP). The energy used in our bodies is released as a result of the breakdown of the ATP molecule:

$$ATP \xrightarrow{\text{breakdown}} energy$$

Virtually all energy used by the cells in the body is based on ATP and the more energy used the more ATP is needed. The body only contains enough ATP for about 10 seconds of maximal movement, and so it has to produce fresh supplies of ATP from energy stores obtained from nutrients (fig 5).

As the concentration of ATP in skeletal muscle is relatively low, another substance, creatine phosphate, acts as the immediate energy source for a short time during the initial burst of contractile activity. However, the amount of creatine phosphate is limited and when muscular activity is to be maintained for any length of time ATP must be produced from the Krebs cycle and glycolytic reactions.

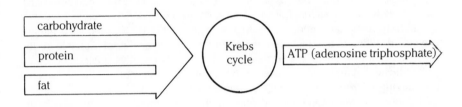

Fig 5 *Energy conversion*

The breakdown mechanism for each of the three energy nutrients is different. There are differences in the way these nutrients are stored in the body and also in the way they are taken out of storage and broken down to ATP, and these differences become very important in sport. This is because both the kind of exercise and the intensity of the energy demand affect how the nutrients will be used.

The primary function of carbohydrate is as a source of energy and so it is mobilised as soon as ATP is needed. Carbohydrates are stored in the liver and muscles in the form of glycogen. When energy is needed the glycogen is taken from storage and broken down to smaller glucose molecules. The way this glucose is converted to energy depends upon the kind of exercise. Anaerobic exercise, which is often described as short maximal effort activity, requires energy breakdown even though there is little or no oxygen in the muscles for combustion.

The scarcity of oxygen makes it less efficient for the body to use its glycogen fuel source for energy, but the glycogen can be broken down incompletely to provide energy even without oxygen. If this happens the end product is lactic acid which is the well-known cause of burning muscles and fatigue. If oxygen is available in sufficient quantities the breakdown of glycogen can continue via Krebs cycle to the production of ATP. This is known as aerobic exercise and the energy yield from this is approximately 300 times greater than anaerobic activity (fig 6).

As glycogen can be broken down for energy whether or not oxygen is present, carbohydrate is the most versatile nutrient. When glycogen stores become diminished or when exercise continues for some time, fat is the next energy nutrient to be mobilised from storage. Fat can only be broken down in the presence of oxygen. Different metabolic processes are involved and fats require 13 per cent more oxygen for their oxidation than carbohydrates.

As fats yield more than twice as many calories as an equivalent weight of protein or carbohydrate they are a very concentrated form of energy. 454 g (1 lb) of pure fat will contribute just over 4000 kcal, or the equivalent of a whole day's energy requirement for an athlete in training. Fat normally makes up between 15 and 20 per cent of the body weight, with women on average having a higher content than men. In some obese people it can comprise up to 40 per cent of body weight. This large amount of fat stored in the body gives it a virtually unlimited fuel source in exercise.

The primary function of protein is not as an energy source. The main roles of protein are to replace cells, build new tissue and as a component of enzymes and hormones. As it is needed for these functions it is not normally converted to energy. But recent research suggests that amino acids from protein are oxidised during periods of intense exercise resulting in a reduction in the size of the amino acid pool available for the synthesis of body tissue. The reasons for this have not been fully explained but could well indicate that a higher-than-average intake of protein may be required by people undertaking an arduous programme of training or sport.

The fourth source of energy and one which is becoming more common in the affluent western world is alcohol with 1 g of pure alcohol yielding 7 kcal (29 kJ).

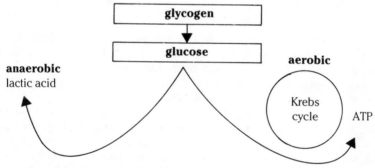

Fig 6   *Carbohydrate metabolism*

Fatigue

Fatigue is the inability to maintain a given exercise intensity and can be simply explained as an imbalance between the rates of ATP utilisation and replenishment at the skeletal muscle. During prolonged exercise, fatigue is mainly the result of the muscle glycogen stores decreasing to levels which cannot support the rate of ATP resynthesis demanded by the exercise intensity. If the glycogen concentration in the skeletal muscle is increased above normal levels it can be shown that glycogen depletion and the onset of fatigue can be delayed during prolonged heavy exercise.

When the muscles become fully depleted of glycogen as a result of intense, continuous exercise, it can take up to 40 hours for them to return to their normal glycogen levels even if a high carbohydrate diet is consumed. Extreme cases have been reported where glycogen levels have not totally replenished after seven days.

The reason for this long period of glycogen resynthesis in the muscle is being attributed in part to the development of trauma and damage in the muscle cells from the intense exercise resulting in a slowing-down of the biochemical reactions. It also appears that the more a muscle is worked during training the more adaptation takes place with a consequent improvement in synthesis rate.

The amount of carbohydrate in the diet affects the rate of glycogen resynthesis, and a high carbohydrate diet is needed to keep muscle glycogen levels high during continuous training. The amount of carbohydrate necessary to maintain the muscle glycogen levels is considered to be between 400 and 600 g per day, and a diet containing 200 g or less of carbohydrate has little or no effect on muscle glycogen storage over a 24-hour period.

Glycogen storage in the liver takes precedence over muscle storage and one high-carbohydrate meal is sufficient to replenish all liver glycogen losses.

There is a significant difference in the glycogen stores of a trained athlete and a person who has not undertaken a programme of training, with the trained athlete having up to twice as much glycogen available in the muscles. The well-nourished, trained athlete will also have higher levels of glycogen in the liver.

Improving performance

It is possible to increase the muscle glycogen above the normal resting values by first depleting the stores in the muscle by exercise and then consuming a diet rich in carbohydrate. This is called 'glycogen supercompensation', and although it has not been shown to increase running speed it allows an athlete to maintain a selected running speed for a longer period so that the overall time is improved.

During exercise the oxidation of fats contributes to energy production but cannot normally be metabolised sufficiently rapidly to cover the muscles' needs without some contribution from carbohydrates. However, fat utilisation helps to extend limited carbohydrate stores. The onset of fatigue has been shown to happen much earlier when fat forms a large proportion of the energy in the diet.

Training increases the aerobic capacity of the muscles and also their ability to metabolise fat. From current research it seems that the most effective method of delaying the onset of fatigue during prolonged exercise is a combination of training and a controlled increase in carbohydrate consumption. The carbohydrate should not be taken immediately before the exercise as this hinders the breakdown of fats and as a consequence gives a more rapid decrease in muscle glycogen.

The composition of the diet is critical to performance and dietary intake can be manipulated to optimise glycogen stores. Since the work of Bergstrom and Huttman in the 1960s, which outlined the initial concepts, a technique has been developed to increase the glycogen stores in the muscles and liver by a combination of dietary modification and exercise. This technique, which now has many variations, is called 'carbohydrate loading' and its theory and application are discussed in more detail in chapter 12.

5 Energy requirements

Energy is used every second of our lives. Even during sleep there are vast numbers of chemical and physical activities taking place in the cells and organs.

The body's activities which take place when you are at rest are known as the basal metabolism ('metabolism' is a general term to cover all the chemical changes occurring in the body). This basal metabolism in adults amounts to between 1200 and 1800 kcal (5000 to 7500 kJ) per day. The basal metabolic rate (BMR) is comparatively constant for individuals but can vary widely between different people. The main factors determining the basal metabolic energy requirements are body size, age, sex and the secretions from the endocrine glands. The metabolic rate is usually higher in males that females.

Over 50 per cent of the BMR is expended in the brain and liver (table 6).

A number of other factors besides the BMR have to be taken into consideration before the total energy requirement can be determined. These requirements can be defined in the following categories:

specific nutrient metabolism

effects of climate

occupational requirements

training (quantity, frequency and intensity)

sport participation.

Energy is expended during the digestion and absorption of food. The actual amount of

Table 6   *Percentage of basal metabolic rate (BMR) due to the five major organs and the rest of the body*

| Organ | Organ weight (kg) | Organ metabolism | |
		kcal/day	BMR (%)
brain	1.4	365	21
heart	0.3	180	10
kidneys	0.3	120	7
liver	1.6	560	32
lungs	0.8	160	9
all others	65.6	395	21

These figures represent a 70 kg (154 lb) adult male with a BMR of 1780 kcal/day.

(Adapted from Briggs and Calloway 1979)

energy used varies with the food source, but if the diet contains a great deal of meat the increase of energy requirement over the BMR may be as high as 18 per cent. Normally the energy expenditure on digestion of food is estimated at beween 6 and 10 per cent of the BMR.

Humans, being warm-blooded animals, possess heat-regulating processes which keep the body temperature constant. Energy is used in keeping the body temperature constant in both hot and cold environments.

Occupational requirements can vary widely depending upon the amount of physical activity needed in the job. Examples of occupational energy usage are given in table 7.

Table 7   *Occupational energy expenditure*

Work	Average energy expenditure	
	kJ/minute	*kcal/minute*
Light		
most domestic work		
lorry driving		
light industrial and assembly	10–20	2.5–4.9
carpentry, bricklaying		
Moderate		
non-mechanised agricultural		
digging, shovelling	21–30	5.0–7.4
Strenuous		
coal mining		
steel furnace work	over 30	over 7.5

The energy requirement of people doing sports is determined by the type of sporting activity; and in any sport a major expenditure of energy happens during training.

The most demanding are the endurance sports. It has been estimated that at the extreme end of the scale the energy cost for athletes running 250 km in 24 hours was 18 600 kcal (77.8 MJ). Typical energy expenditures for different types of sport are given in table 8.

Research also shows that energy consumption increases rapidly with increasing intensity of activity. So at a slow run of 3.3 metres per second (m/s), a person would consume about 10.8 kcal per kg of body weight per hour. If the running speed is doubled to 6.6 m/s energy utilisation increases to 85 kcal. As running speed doubles, energy requirements increase eightfold. The same relationship between exercise intensity and energy expenditure is found in all other sports.

Table 8 *Energy expenditure in sport*

Sport	Rate/speed	Approximate expenditure per minute for a 70 kg person	
		kcal	*kJ*
running	3.3 m/s	12.6	53.0
	5.0 m/s	17.5	73.0
	6.6 m/s	99.2	415.0
swimming	0.17 m/s	3.5	14.6
	0.9 m/s	14.7	61.5
	1.16 m/s	30.1	126.0
cycling	10 km/hour	5.0	21.0
	20 km/hour	10.0	42.0
rowing	0.84 m/s	3.2	13.4
	1.6 m/s	12.7	53.1
gymnastics	light	3.5	14.6
	competition	17.5	73.0
throwing	training	12.8	53.5
fencing	–	10.5	44.0
skiing	3.8 m/s	18.0	75.3
table tennis	–	5.25	22.0

Females have on average an energy requirement about 10 per cent lower than males in a comparable performance.

During aerobic exercise an average of 5 kcal is derived from food for every litre of oxygen assimilated by the body. On this basis an athlete with a maximum oxygen capacity of 5 litres per minute can obtain about 25 kcal per minute of aerobic energy. But it is unlikely that the maximum oxygen capacity can be sustained for very long and a value of 70 to 80 per cent of maximum is more realistic. If the oxygen capacity is known you may predict the energy requirement for the exercise. For example, a runner with a 5 litre maximum capapcity running at 75 per cent of that capacity would need between 1000 and 1150 kcal per hour.

Training and competition energy needs are cumulative on other needs; for many athletes this means they would need between 3000 and 6000 kcal per day.

Balancing the diet

It is often difficult to judge whether energy intake balances energy expenditure. A simple way to check is by weighing every day, at the same time of day. If body weight remains constant, then energy balance is about right. A slow gain in weight can indicate excessive intake and a slow loss excessive utilisation.

In addition to total energy intake it is important that the correct balance of energy nutrients is obtained from the diet. The calculation of this nutrient balance is often difficult to understand; nutritionists tend to consider the energy contributed by carbohydrates, fats and proteins as percentages of the total energy intake. So the American College of Sports Medicine's general recommendation for energy nutrient

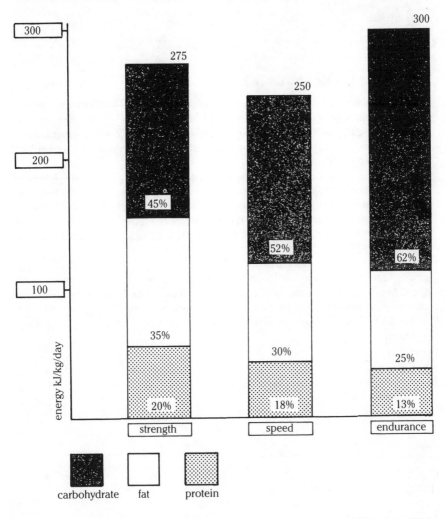

(Adapted from Müller–Wohlfahrt, Montag and Diebschlag 1984)

Fig 7   *Nutrient balances for different sports*

25

balance for athletes is to obtain between 50 and 60 per cent of energy from carbohydrate, 30 to 35 per cent as fat and 10 to 15 per cent as protein. To convert these figures into food intake use the conversion factors for the energy content of nutrients given on page 18.

If these factors are used, calculations for each 1000 calories can be made like this:

Nutrient	Recommended per cent of total	Calories per g	Actual weight in food (g/dry weight)
carbohydrate	50	3.75	133.30
fat	35	9.00	38.90
protein	15	4.00	37.50
total	100 per cent		209.70 g

On this basis, for each 1000 calories a person must eat 133 g (4¾ oz) of carbohydrates such as starches or sugars, 39 g (1⅓ oz) of fats, and 38 g (1⅓ oz) of protein. To complete the exercise use food composition tables (examples given in appendix 2) to build up a series of meals using the ratios of the energy nutrients that we have calculated in the table above.

Whilst the recommended percentages of energy nutrients given by the American College of Sports Medicine are designed to cover most sports, some workers have developed more detailed recommendations for specific sports. These normally require a greater intake of protein for the sports requiring strength, and higher carbohydrate intake for endurance sports. An example of these different requirements is given in fig 7.

It would be nice to be able to define precise nutrient requirements for each sport or group of sports in this way. But in practice it is almost impossible to achieve these fine distinctions in nutrient content from day to day, and on balance evidence suggests that athletes who have followed the general guidelines have obtained just as much benefit as those who have suffered the inconvenience, and often the expense, of proprietary regimens.

6 Vitamins in sport

A considerable and unfortunate mythology has for a number of years surrounded the role of vitamins in sport. In their search for the magic ingredient which will dramatically improve their performance, many athletes have been tempted to consume large quantities of vitamins. In addition many vitamins have had functions attributed to them which do not stand up to strict scientific scrutiny.

The high energy expenditure of athletes means that their requirements of certain vitamins will be higher than those of the average person, and it is important that these increased needs are met from the diet. If there is a risk that the chosen diet will not supply these additional requirements, a good-quality vitamin supplement can be added as a form of nutritional insurance.

If supplements are taken, the amounts consumed should bear a relationship to the individual's daily needs. Excessive consumption of any single vitamin should be avoided.

As we described in chapter 2, vitamins are organic compounds essential for life. They are compounds which, although required by the body in minute amounts, perform specific and vital functions in the cells and tissues. They cannot be synthesised by the body and their absence or improper absorption results in specific deficiency diseases.

The 13 compounds classed as vitamins for people differ from each other in physiological function, chemical structure and distribution in food. The principal functions of these vitamins are outlined in appendix 1.

A number of other sustances have over the years been described as vitamins, but these have not met the strict criteria of being proven essential for human life and therefore cannot be considered to be vitamins. Examples are choline, inositol and para-aminobenzoic acid (PABA), which are compounds that have been shown to be needed by some other animal species but whose requirement by humans has not been proven. Two other compounds, laetrile and pangamic acid have been marketed as vitamin B_{17} and B_{15} respectively. There is no scientific basis for this classification and sale of laetrile has been restricted in a number of countries due to potential toxicity.

The 13 recognised vitamins are grouped according to solubility. Vitamins A, D, E and K are fat-soluble and form one group, whilst the eight vitamins of the B-complex group and vitamin C are water-soluble. As the water-soluble vitamins cannot be stored in the body in appreciable amounts, they have to be taken in regularly. Any intake of these water-soluble vitamins in excess of the body's immediate needs is likely to be excreted in the urine.

The B-complex vitamins are of importance in sports nutrition as they are all vital components of major co-enzymes in the body and as a group they play many diverse roles in energy metabolism.

In general the requirements of the B-complex vitamins appear to be related to calorie intake up to about 5000 calories per day, and on this basis athletes can be expected to need at least double the recommended daily amounts of these vitamins.

27

A number of studies have shown that a deficiency of the B-complex vitamins over a period of a few weeks will lead to a decrease in endurance capacity.

We will now look at the roles of the individual vitamins in the context of sports nutrition.

Vitamin B_1 (thiamin)

This is an active part of the co-enzyme thiamin pyrophosphate which is known to be necessary for at least four enzyme systems and is intimately bound up in carbohydrate metabolism.

The body's need for thiamin is dependent upon energy expenditure and is also influenced by carbohydrate consumption. Daily requirements for thiamin are based on carbohydrate intake, and the United Kingdom recommendations are based on 96 μg thiamin/MJ (0.4 mg/1000 kcal). In the USA the amount recommended by the National Academy of Sciences is 0.5 mg/1000 kcal. As the calorie intake of athletes is well above that of the average person, the thiamin levels must be increased correspondingly. There is some evidence that thiamin excretion increases during regular intensive exercise such as training although the causes have not been fully identified.

Vitamin B_2 (riboflavin)

In the form of the phosphate ester, this acts as a co-enzyme of the flavin enzymes concerned with hydrogen transfer. These flavin enzymes of the respiratory chain intervene in the general metabolism of carbohydrates, amino acids and fatty acids. Some people have suggested that riboflavin is, because of its functions, important for endurance type sports and also for the functioning of the glycolytic enzymes. If this is true, a deficiency could have a negative effect on anaerobic activity where a high glycolytic rate is important.

The British recommendation for vitamin B_2 is 240 μg/MJ (1 mg/1000 kcal) of resting metabolism whereas the Americans have a recommended intake of 0.6 mg/1000 kcal of total energy utilisation.

Niacin (nicotinic acid or nicotinamide)

This acts as a component of two co-enzymes concerned with tissue respiration, fat synthesis and glycolysis. Whilst most B vitamins show an increased need with increasing energy consumption, there appears to be an upper limit for niacin. Nicotinic acid can inhibit the mobilisation of free fatty acids and this could impede performance by forcing more rapid consumption of glycogen by the muscles.

The human body is capable of forming nicotinic acid from the amino acid tryptophan. Under normal conditions however the amounts of nicotinic acid formed this way are inadequate to meet the total daily requirement and the balance must be obtained from food sources. The United Kingdom recommendation for niacin is 2.7 mg nicotinic acid equivalent/MJ or 11.3 mg/1000 kcal of resting metabolism. The American National Academy of Sciences recommendations are much higher with a requirement of 6.6 mg niacin equivalent/1000 kcal of total energy utilisation.

Vitamin B₆ (pyridoxine)

This acts as a co-enzyme of over 60 enzymes and plays a central role in the biochemical reactions whereby nutrient amino acids are converted into the particular amino acids required by the cells. Vitamin B_6 is also involved in the initial breakdown of glycogen. The intimate involvement of vitamin B_6 in amino acid metabolism means that an increase in dietary protein leads to increased vitamin B_6 requirements.

Vitamin B₁₂ (cyanocobalamin)

This is involved in a variety of processes including carbohydrate and fat metabolism. It has become a popular vitamin for supplementation by athletes, often by injection, although most studies have shown no added benefit where a B_{12} deficiency does not exist.

Vitamin B_{12} plays a role in preventing pernicious anaemia.

Pantothenic acid

This is part of co-enzyme A and plays a part in the intermediate stages of carbohydrate and fat metabolism leading to energy release. It is also involved in the synthesis of amino acids, fatty acids, sterols and steroid hormones.

There have been a number of studies which suggest that supplementation with pantothenic acid is beneficial to physical activity. But more detailed experimentation is needed before these theories can be confirmed.

Folic acid (folacin)

This is related to DNA synthesis and a deficiency may lead to anaemia. To date, little work has been carried out on the effects of folic acid on physical performance, although theoretically a deficiency in folic acid could affect an endurance athlete due to anaemic effects upon oxygen transport.

Biotin

Biotin plays a number of roles in the metabolism. It acts as a co-enzyme in the formation and oxidation of fats and proteins including the maintenance of normal blood glucose concentrations from fat and protein whenever the carbohydrate intake from food becomes insufficient.

There is also some evidence that biotin is necessary for the utilisation of vitamin B_{12}.

Biotin is produced by bacteria normally present in the intestines. Certain proteins including one found in raw egg white can bind up biotin and make it unavailable to the body, but biotin deficiencies are very rare in humans.

Vitamin C (ascorbic acid)

This is a water-soluble vitamin, essential for the formation of collagen (a major component of connective tissue) and also for the maintenance of the normal function of these tissues. Vitamin C also exerts a stimulant action on the defensive mechanisms of the body. It has a variety of roles and some specific functions are still not fully understood. Vitamin C has also been shown to be an important component in the absorption of iron from non-animal sources.

There are some studies which indicate that vitamin C needs are increased under conditions of extreme athletic stress and that vitamin C requirements also increase at higher temperatures. As normal body temperature increases under intense stress, some workers consider the vitamin C requirements of athletes to be many times higher than the United Kingdom recommended daily amount of 30 mg per day.

Athletes should also take into consideration the positive effect of vitamin C on iron absorption as low iron levels are commonly found in both male and female athletes during training.

Vitamin A

A term used to designate several related compounds which are biologically active. These compounds exist either as preformed vitamin A (retinol, vitamin A acetate or palmitate, and retinoic acid), or as substances which can be converted into vitamin A by the body called provitamins. A number of forms of provitamin A are found amongst the yellow carotenoid plant pigments such as beta-carotene, which is a carotenoid found in many dark green and deep yellow fruits and vegetables and which has the highest biological activity of the carotenes. When the beta-carotene molecule is taken into the body it can be converted into vitamin A and the main site of this conversion in humans appears to be in the intestinal wall. Beta-carotene is considered to be a safe way of taking in vitamin A as the body only converts it when needed and as a result beta-carotene does not appear to cause the adverse effects associated with retinol as a source of vitamin A activity. Beta-carotene is also thought to have a number of other functions and research is being carried out into its effects on the reduction of the rates of development of cancer in certain body tissues.

Very large continuous intakes of vitamin A as retinol or its esters are known to be toxic. Whilst the toxic levels are many times the normal daily intake taken over a long period of time (for example intakes in excess of 50 000 IU a day for number of months), it is generally recommended that the intake of vitamin A, particularly in the form of supplements, should be kept below 10 000 IU a day.

One documented case of vitamin A toxicity is that of a 15-year-old male football player who consumed over 100 000 IU of vitamin A a day in cod liver oil, liver, milk and vitamin supplements. He took this diet for over two months in a misguided attempt to improve his performance. The result was a stiffness and swelling in his legs with structural changes taking place in the long bones (periosteal ossification). The symptoms cleared within a month of the diet being discontinued.

Vitamin A plays an important role in the visual processes as it forms part of the pigment in the retina of the eye which converts light to nerve impulses. It is also involved in the formation and maintenance of the epithelial tissues which seal the body from infection, such as the skin, and mucous linings of the mouth, stomach and genital tracts. A deficiency of vitamin A can manifest itself as temporary night blindness or a loss of resistance to infection.

Vitamin D

This is involved in regulating calcium and phosphorus metabolism during the formation of bones and teeth. Its special function is to make these two minerals available in the blood which constantly bathes the bones so that they can be deposited on the bone mass. This is a constant process throughout life as the bone mass is always changing.

Vitamin D can be made in the human body when the ultraviolet light from the sun interacts with a derivative of cholesterol in the skin.

Dietary vitamin D is necessary when there is a reduction in the amount of sunlight or in the amount of exposed skin, for example in winter in the United Kingdom when not only is the sunlight reduced, but people tend to cover almost all of their bodies.

As with vitamin A, vitamin D can be toxic if consumed in large quantities over a long period of time. If vitamin D fortified foods or supplements are taken the total intake should not exceed 400 IU (10 μg) a day.

Vitamin E

Vitamin E is in fact the generic name given to a series of chemically related compounds called tocopherols. The major function of vitamin E is as an anti-oxidant in preventing harmful oxidation of fatty acids. It also helps to maintain capillary and blood platelet tonicity. Some studies on vitamin E in sport appear to indicate a higher-than-average need for athletes undergoing the stress of training and competitions. One study on the effects of vitamin E supplementation on performance at high altitudes showed that subjects receiving 1200 IU of vitamin E a day had an increased endurance and reduced oxygen debt.

Vitamin K

This has an important role in regulating blood coagulation and occurs in a number of forms. It is found in green leafy vegetables and some vegetable oils. As about half the human vitamin K requirement is derived from bacterial synthesis in the intestines, the amount required from the diet is relatively low, and it is a vitamin which is very rarely supplemented.

7 Minerals in sport

The human body must obtain all the minerals it needs from food and water. As we described in chapter 2, the minerals required fall into two groups classified by the amounts needed. These are

macro minerals – those which are required in relatively large amounts (up to grammes per day)

trace minerals – those which are only required in minute amounts (milligrammes or microgrammes per day).

Regular, consistent intake of both groups of minerals is important for athletes as large losses can occur during strenuous exercise.

One of the reasons for this is that body fluids consist mainly of water in which inorganic salts, protein and some organic compounds are dissolved. Inorganic salts belong to a class of substances known as electrolytes. When dissolved in water the molecules of electrolytes separate into two or more electrically charged particles called ions. Salts, acids and bases are electrolytes while compounds such as glucose, protein and urea are not because they are molecules that do not ionise.

Ions which carry a positive charge are called cations and those with a negative charge anions. The ionisation of sodium chloride (table salt) can be represented as:

$$NaCl \rightleftharpoons Na^+ + Cl^-$$
$$\text{salt} \qquad \text{cation} + \text{anion}$$

The main cationic electrolytes in the body fluids are sodium, potassium, magnesium and calcium. The principal anion is chloride with smaller amounts of sulphate, carbonate and phosphate also being present (table 9). Electrical balance is always maintained in the fluid compartments of the body. As a measure of the total combining power of electrolytes in solution, a unit of measure which is related to the number of electrical charges carried by the ions present in the solution must be used. This unit of measure is milli-equivalents (mEq). The cations and anions in each fluid compartment of the body, as measured in milli-equivalents, are equal.

Electrolytes play an important part in maintaining the acid-base balance of the blood and tissues, and the maintenance of balance is a function of normal metabolism. Blood is slightly alkaline in the pH range 7.3 to 7.45 and varies only within narrow limits.

All water lost by the body, except that associated with expiration of air from the lungs, is accompanied by electrolytes, mainly sodium and chloride. During strenuous physical exercise the main source of electrolyte loss is through sweat. Between 2.3 and 3.4 g of sodium chloride (salt) are lost in each litre of sweat.

If, in the case of high sweat loss, only water is replaced, the electrolyte concentrations in the body's extracellular fluid become out of balance and the extracellular fluid can become more dilute than normal. If this happens water will move from the dilute extracellular fluid to the more concentrated intracellular fluid by

Table 9 *Relative amounts of the principal electrolytes in blood and sweat*

	Mineral content (g/l)	
	Blood	Sweat
sodium (Na$^+$)	3.2	1.2
chloride (Cl$^-$)	3.6	1.4
potassium (K$^+$)	0.2	0.2
magnesium (Mg$^+$)	0.02	0.04
total	7.02	2.84

a process known as osmosis, and potassium will move from the intracellular fluid to the extracellular fluid. When this happens the cells become overhydrated and cramps may develop because of salt depletion.

If only part of the water and none of the salt is replaced the extracellular fluid volume will fall. If this loss of volume is severe the blood pressure will also fall to the point of producing faintness. In very severe cases this can produce circulatory failure.

It is essential that electrolyte losses as well as water losses are replaced after exercise. This can be accomplished by frequently drinking vegetable or fruit juices, proprietary electrolyte replacement drinks or, if these are not available, by adding small quantities of salt to the water.

In addition to the macro minerals for maintaining the electrolyte balance, calcium, magnesium and phosphorus are needed continuously for the growth and repair of structures such as bones and teeth.

Calcium

Calcium is the major mineral component of the body and over 1 kg is contained in the average adult. All but about 1 per cent of the body's calcium is found in the bones and teeth.

Calcium balance has recently been shown to be more critical than originally thought. Bone mass is not static but undergoes a continuous turnover throughout life, reaching a peak mass at about the age of 35 and then declining. It declines very rapidly in women for about three to seven years after menopause resulting in a less dense bone structure. This condition, known as osteoporosis, may lead to bone fractures in the elderly, and fractures of the vertebrae and hips are among the important manifestations of osteoporosis. Women have more tendency to fracture than men.

Recent studies indicate that the daily requirement of calcium may be considerably higher than the 500 mg per day which is the United Kingdom recommended daily amount (RDA). In the USA the RDA is 800 mg and some authorities are now considering a requirement of 1000 mg a day for premenopausal women and elderly men and 1500 mg a day for postmenopausal women. Women should start to take these higher levels well before the onset of the menopause.

Consistent higher-than-average exercise and activity appears to slow down the rate of bone loss. The major risk is to female athletes who retire from their sport in their late thirties or early forties and significantly reduce their level of exercise.

Not all the calcium in foods is available to the body, and only about 20 to 40 per cent of the calcium consumed is absorbed from the intestinal tract into the bloodstream. Many things affect the absorption of calcium, including the vitamin D status of the body, the pH of the upper intestinal tract, the presence of phytates (phosphorus compounds found in cereals) and the amount of fat in the diet.

High protein intakes can lead to the increased excretion of calcium in the urine and faeces. This is very important for athletes on high-protein and high-calorie diets as they

Table 10   *Foods containing high calcium levels*

	Calcium content	
Food	mg/oz	mg/100 g
parmesan cheese	346	1220
fried whitebait	244	860
cheddar cheese	227	800
edam cheese	210	740
fried sprats	201	710
spinach, boiled	170	600
sardines, canned in oil	156	550
black treacle	142	500
condensed milk, whole, sweetened	107	380
canned pilchards in tomato sauce	85	300
figs, dried raw	79	280
almonds	71	250
low-fat soya flour	68	240
watercress, raw	62	220
muesli (average value)	57	200
natural yoghurt	51	180
white flour (fortified)	39	138
liquid skimmed milk	37	130
liquid whole milk	34	120

(From Paul and Southgate 1978)

will need to increase their intake of calcium. For example, in a high-calorie diet of about 5000 kcal per day of which protein comprises 15 per cent, the protein intake will be in the region of 185 g. As this protein level is about two and a half times the United Kingdom RDA for men, the calcium intake needs to be substantially increased; a daily intake of 1500 mg per day would not be unreasonable. Examples of foods containing high calcium levels are given in table 10.

Iron

This is another mineral critical to the nutrition of athletes, and many investigations have been carried out into the iron status of athletes undergoing rigorous training.

Anaemia is a condition characterised by a lower-than-normal concentration of haemoglobin in the blood. Haemoglobin is a red compound consisting of a protein called globin connected to a substance called haem which contains iron in the ferrous state. The body of a healthy adult contains between 3 and 4 g of iron, and about 65 to 70 per cent of this iron is present in the haemoglobin.

Since haemoglobin plays a central part in the blood's oxygen transport function (one molecule of haemoglobin can carry four molecules of oxygen), anaemia can reduce oxygen delivery to body tissues.

In recent years there have been numerous reports of anaemia in athletes, particularly those in endurance sports, and the term 'sports anaemia' has been coined to identify this condition. As anaemia can have a significant effect on maximum performance, 'sports anaemia' has recently become an area of concern in sports medicine.

Whilst the incidence of clinical-grade anaemia is quite low, a substantial percentage of athletes, particularly those in endurance sports, show haemoglobin concentrations on the low side. In addition many athletes manifest low iron stores and therefore are at an increased risk of developing anaemia.

It has also been observed that a transient anaemia may occur at the onset of heavy training, but the mechanism which causes this is not fully understood.

Female athletes who have heavy menstrual losses can be at risk of iron deficiency during periods of heavy training.

Absorption of iron is a complex process influenced by the type of iron obtained from the diet. There are also a number of dietary factors which make iron more or less available for the body to use. Normally only about one-tenth of the dietary iron is absorbed by the body.

Two types of iron are found in the diet and these are known as haem iron and non-haem iron. About 40 per cent of the iron in animal tissue is haem iron and is available in a form that the body can readily absorb. The remaining iron in animal tissue and the iron in dairy products and non-animal sources (eg vegetables and grains) is non-haem iron and is more difficult to absorb.

Iron absorption is further decreased in diets which include tea, coffee or whole grains, as the phytates in the grains and tannins in tea and coffee can form compounds with non-haem iron making absorption difficult. Vitamin C and animal protein help to increase the absorption of non-haem iron from foods.

Teenagers of both sexes tend to have higher iron needs than adults as the blood supplies and iron reserves expand during this period of rapid growth, and a higher level of iron intake is required to maintain normal haemoglobin levels and build reserves. Examples of foods containing high levels of iron are shown in table 11.

Table 11 *Foods containing high iron levels*

| Food | Iron content | |
	mg/oz	mg/100 g
cockles, boiled	7.6	26.0
black pudding	5.7	20.0
roast pigeon	5.5	19.4
pig liver, stewed	4.8	17.0
lamb kidney, fried	3.4	12.0
lamb liver, stewed	2.8	10.0
black treacle	2.6	9.2
soya flour (low fat)	2.6	9.1
roast pheasant	2.4	8.4
roast partridge	2.2	7.7
ox heart, stewed	2.2	7.7
egg yolk, raw	1.7	6.1
oysters	1.7	6.0
mussels	1.6	5.8
almonds	1.2	4.2
figs, dried	1.2	4.2
apricots, dried	1.2	4.1
spinach, boiled	1.1	4.0
grilled lean steak	1.0	3.4

(From Paul and Southgate 1978)

Trace minerals

The essential trace minerals are required by the body in such small amounts (mg or μg) that it is easy to underestimate their importance in nutrition. As with vitamins, the body cannot maintain a healthy condition without them.

Trace minerals can be found in catalytic or structural roles in enzymes, vitamins and hormones and this is why such tiny amounts have a profound effect on the body. For example, chromium is associated with glucose metabolism, probably as a co-factor for insulin, and it is thought that one single atom of chromium can trigger the action of insulin in an individual cell.

Copper is essential for the mobilisation of iron in the synthesis of haemoglobin and is also a constituent of many enzymes that function in tissue metabolism. Copper is essential to prevent anaemia, even in the presence of adequate supplies of iron. Manganese is an important element believed to be involved in the synthesis of cartilage. Manganese is also found in many enzyme systems.

Zinc is known to be part of the structure of at least 70 enzymes. As part of the enzyme collagenase it is involved in the synthesis of collagen, the protein that binds cells to form tissues. It is also required for the maintenance of the natural system of immunity to inflammation and infection and for the maintenance of normal taste acuity and appetite. Zinc is responsible for the healthy growth and functioning of the reproductive system in both sexes. Zinc is lost in sweat and studies on the serum zinc levels in a number of long-distance runners showed that they were on the extreme lower level of normal.

Selenium is a recently recognised trace mineral; it was only in 1957 that researchers discovered that a mineral which was once thought to be highly toxic was as vital to the diet as iron, zinc or copper.

Although the functions of selenium are closely related to vitamin E, selenium has specific anti-oxidant properties of its own, particularly in protecting tissues of the vital organs such as the liver, heart and lungs. Most dietary selenium is obtained from animal protein sources, mainly organ meats. It also occurs to a lesser extent in vegetables and fruits such as potatoes, maize, pears and peaches. Vitamin E and selenium act together in the body to control harmful tissue oxidation which occurs particularly when the body is stressed, for example in sports participation. When vitamin E and selenium are together they act synergistically, which means that their combined effect is greater than the effect of the same amounts of each nutrient acting alone.

Iodine is an essential constituent of hormones produced by the thyroid gland in the neck. Deficiency causes this gland to enlarge to give a condition known as goitre.

The area of trace mineral research is one of the most interesting in nutritional science. A few minerals such as iron, iodine and zinc have been studied for a long time and appear to have well-defined human requirements. The next category are those minerals which can be shown to be associated with essential bodily functions in humans and have only recently had their requirements established. These are chromium, copper, manganese, molybdenum, selenium and fluorine.

A third category comprises minerals which are required for other animal species but where their function in humans is still unclear at the present level of knowledge. This group includes tin, nickel, silicon and vanadium. But it is typical that a trace element which plays an essential role for one or more mammals will eventually prove to be essential for people too.

8 Fluid balance, temperature regulation and electrolytes

Each cell of a complex multicellular organism such as a human being is surrounded by a fluid called extracellular fluid (ie fluid outside the cell). This fluid, the body's internal environment, acts as the medium for exchange of nutrients and waste products and provides the stable physiochemical environment for membrane and cell function. The ability of the body to maintain a relatively constant volume and level of constituents of this internal environment is basic for survival. The maintenance of this constant environment is called homeostasis.

To understand this more clearly, imagine that the body is a tank of tropical fish in a large room (fig 8). The fish need an environment with a relatively unchanging temperature, regulated within very narrow limits. The temperature of the water in the tank is maintained by a heater and controlled by a thermostat. When the room cools down, the heater is automatically switched on and reheats the tank water to the desired temperature; if the room temperature rises above that of the water the heater will stop operating.

But the fish not only need a constant water temperature, they also have a requirement with regard to the water's purity. Since the fish excrete waste directly into the water, toxic substances will eventually build up and poison them. This means at least part of the water needs changing at frequent intervals to avoid excessive accumulation of unwanted material.

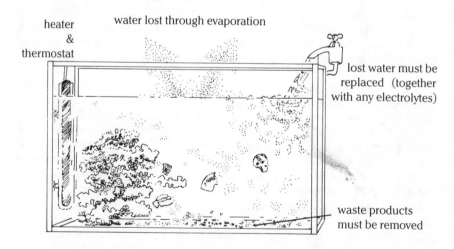

heater & thermostat

water lost through evaporation

lost water must be replaced (together with any electrolytes)

waste products must be removed

Fig 8   *Maintenance of a constant environment is an essential requisite for a healthy fish tank community*

If our imaginary tank contained sea-water fish, their immediate environment would be a complex solution of dissolved minerals and salts, mainly sodium chloride (table salt). As water evaporates from the tank the level of water decreases, while the amount of dissolved salts remains constant; the solution in which the fish are living would become increasingly more concentrated. This would impair their health and eventually kill them. To overcome this, water has to be constantly replaced to maintain the correct volume.

Unfortunately, when the water is changed to remove toxic waste the important salts are also removed. If these are not replenished the solution in the tank will gradually become diluted and upset the constant environment.

For the fish to remain healthy, there must be a constant temperature, a constant volume of water, and a constant concentration of dissolved salts. And so it is with the human body.

The body regulates its internal, or core, temperature by altering blood flow to the skin. The blood transports excess heat to the body's surface where it is dissipated to the outside world by evaporation of sweat. Kidneys control the volume of water and salts by processing the body's fluids and excreting waste products. The levels of water and electrolytes are also regulated by the kidneys. The body also loses water and electrolytes through sweat (part of the heat control system) and pure water through exhaled air from the lungs. These losses must be replaced from the diet (remember the necessary water changes in the fish tank), otherwise there will be severe dehydration and metabolic disturbance.

The most important factors affecting the stability of the body's internal environment are the concentrations of water and electrolytes. Although in practice the fate of water and the electrolytes are interdependent, it is easier to discuss them separately.

Water

Water is by far the most abundant component of animals and in humans it constitutes approximately 60 per cent of total body weight (fig 9). The distribution of this water in the body is given in table 12. There is considerable variation of water content between individuals and the range can be as wide as 40 to 80 per cent depending upon the amount of fat in the body. Since fat tissue contains less water than muscle tissue, the percentage of total body weight which is water is lower in a fat person and higher in a muscular person. So athletes generally will have a higher water content when calculated as a percentage of body weight.

Although not usually regarded as a nutrient, water is vital. It serves as a solvent, and a regulator of body temperature. It carries nutrients to each cell and transports the waste products away. It also works in digestion and is needed for all chemical reactions in metabolism.

It is not surprising then that daily water losses must be replaced through the diet as food and drink. A person's needs will vary depending upon their physiological and climatic conditions. Table 13 shows average figures for water losses and gains in adults.

Exercise increases muscle activity which converts chemical energy into mechanical energy and a by-product of this energy exchange is heat. Most energy conversions

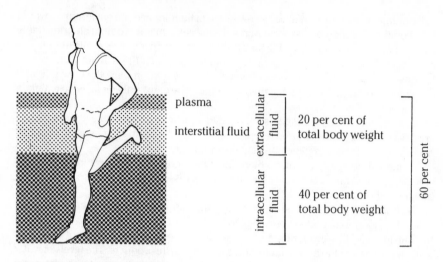

Fig 9   *The distribution of water within the body*

Table 12   *Percentage of the total body water found in the various tissues and organs*

Tissue/organ	Total body weight (%)	Tissue/organ	Total body weight (%)
muscle	50.8	brain	2.7
skeleton	12.5	lungs	2.4
skin	6.6	fatty tissue	2.3
blood	4.7	kidneys	0.6
intestine	3.2	spleen	0.4
liver	2.8	rest of body	11.0
			100.0

generate some (mainly unwanted) heat; for example in an electric light bulb or a car engine. When the body transforms chemical energy, stored in the form of carbohydrates or fat, into mechanical energy, its temperature rises. To avoid overheating, which would cause coma or death, the body activates a limiting mechanism just like the thermostat in the fish tank. This mechanism, triggered by hormones, consists of the excretion of body fluids through skin pores commonly known as sweating. Surface moisture cools the skin due to the physical phenomenon called 'heat of evaporation'. This means that when it changes from liquid to gas, water

Table 13   *Normal routes of water gain and loss in adults*

	ml/day
Intake	
drink	1200
in food	1000
metabolically produced	350
total	2550
Output	
insensible loss (skin and lungs)	900
sweat	50
in faeces	100
in urine	1500
total	2550
Alimentary secretions (almost all reabsorbed)	
saliva	500–1500
gastric juice	2000–3000
pancreatic juice	300–1500
bile	250–1100
intestinal secretions (approximate figures)	3000–3000
total	6050–10100

takes up energy. In the case of sweat it must do so by taking heat from the skin. The discomfort you experience on very humid days is due to the failure of the sweat to evaporate and little heat is transferred from the body. The importance of evaporation means that there is no benefit in changing into a dry shirt, for example in a long tennis match, since this simply impedes the process until the shirt is as wet as before. It is best not to place things in the way of a person's cooling system.

The rate of fluid loss is dependent upon energy expenditure, and the temperature and humidity of the environment. But even at rest the body loses water from the skin and in exhaled breath. Fluid loss during exercise can be very high. For example, a 75 kg (165 lb) person can lose up to 4 per cent of body weight during a game of football or more than 5 per cent of body weight (3.75 l or 6.6 pints) over a marathon (table 14). There have been reports of elite marathon runners losing as much as 5 litres of fluid during a race.

Table 14   *Fluid balance: weight losses by sport (kg)*

running	100 m		0.15
	1000 m		1.50
	marathon		4.00
football			3.00
fencing			1.00
cross-country skiing (10 km)			1.00
basketball			1.70

Table 15   *Adverse effects of dehydration*

Plasma vol. loss (%)	*Body water loss (%)*	*Effect*
1	0.5–1	thirst
4	2	strong thirst, sense of oppression, discomfort
6	3	dry mouth, reduction in urinary output
8	4	increased effort for physical work, flushed skin, nausea, apathy
10	5	difficulty in concentrating
12	6	impairment of exercise temperature regulation, increased pulse and respiratory rates
16	8	dizziness, cyanosis and laboured breathing with exercise, indistinct speech, increasing weakness, mental confusion
20	10	spastic muscles, inability to balance with eyes closed, general incapacity, delirium and wakefulness, swollen tongue
22	11	circulatory insufficiency, marked haemoconcentration and decreased blood volume, failing renal function

(Adapted from Greenleaf 1982)

Shortage of water causes more immediate and more intolerable distress than shortage of food. People completely deprived of water soon feel their mouth dry, complain of thirst, and the craving for fluid rapidly becomes compelling (table 15). As time goes on dryness of the mouth increases, production of saliva ceases, and swallowing of food becomes impossible. Finally, when the water loss is about 8 litres (10 to 11 per cent of body weight), delirium is followed by death. This shows how important it is to replenish water lost during strenuous exercise.

As humans have the capacity to dissipate heat through sweating we are able to perform high-intensity physical exercise for prolonged periods. If sweating was not possible then the body would soon overheat and we would eventually die. Fortunately, fatigue and fainting usually intervene before this happens.

In a temperate environment the primary heat source is the body's metabolism. With only a few minutes of maximum physical exertion it is possible to increase the metabolic rate to about 30 times the basal rate. For most people normal body 'core' temperature is 37.0 °C (98.6 °F). People can die if the temperature drops to 27 °C (80.6 °F); on the other hand an increase to only 42.0 °C (107.6 °F) can also be fatal. So overheating seems to be more critical for survival than overcooling. Although part of the ability to perform high-intensity and long periods of physical exercise is inherited, there is ample evidence that tolerance for higher core temperature and associated enhanced maximal sweating capacity can be induced by training in a hot environment.

Since sweat is derived from the interstitial fluid, the volume of this fluid will decrease during exercise. To combat this loss there is a shift of plasma to the interstitial space in proportion to the increase in systolic blood pressure, which is directly proportional to exercise. The magnitude of the shift increases from about 6 per cent (180 ml) with moderate exercise to about 16 per cent (500 ml) during peak (maximal) exercise. A second and more slowly acting mechanism is the production of water liberated from metabolism of the glycogen during exercise. Oxidation of 500 g of muscle glycogen over a period of four to six hours could produce 1500 ml of water.

Fig 10 shows the effect of water consumption on rectal temperature while walking in the heat. The highest temperature occurred when no water was taken and the lowest temperature when water intake equalled sweat output. With moderate exercise at normal ambient temperature, core temperature rises by 0.1 °C for each 1 per cent decrease in body water content. This relationship can be detected with a loss of only 1 per cent (about 450 ml) of body water which emphasises the sensitivity of the interaction. The main cause of dehydration hyperthermia is reduction in sweating and evaporative heat loss.

Highly trained athletes normally have high sweat loss, and unless the conditions in which they are training are very dry most of the sweat will drip off their bodies and will not evaporate; as a consequence the sweat will not contribute to heat dissipation. The plasma volume will decrease due to the increase in blood pressure and will continue to decrease as long as the sweat loss is greater than fluid intake. This will of course decrease the effectiveness of the cardiovascular system to transport oxygen and decrease the ability of the blood to transport heat from the working muscles to the skin. Even a sufficient volume of sweat on the skin cannot dissipate heat that does not arrive

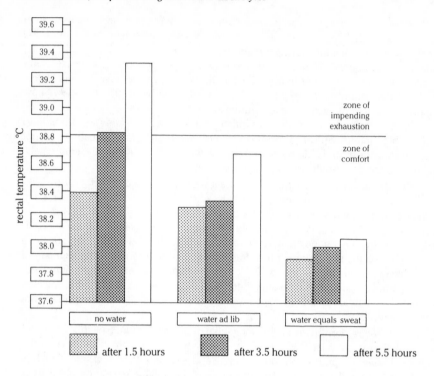

Conditions: walking up a 2.5% grade at 3.5 mph in the heat (T_a = 37.7 °C, rh = 40%).

Fig 10   *Effect of water consumption on body temperature*

at the surface.

No matter how the plasma volume is depleted, and even sitting relatively still for one hour can result in a decrease in plasma volume, an underfilled circulatory system will reduce its volume by vascoconstriction (ie the body narrows the calibre of small blood vessels reducing the amount of blood that can flow through them). Since the working muscles will take priority for the remaining blood plasma, this will further reduce heat transfer and heat dissipation, resulting in a rise in core temperature. The outcome will be heat exhaustion and fainting. A failure to replace needed fluids will only hasten deterioration of physical and mental performance. In fact, people undergoing intensive exercise will require progressively greater fluid intake to compensate for the increased sweating that results from the training.

A classic case of heat exhaustion was experienced by the Italian, Pietro Dorando, who collapsed and had to be helped over the finishing line (he was later disqualified) in the marathon at the 1908 London Olympics. Olympic deaths also happened during the marathon race in the 1912 Stockholm Olympics and in the 100 km cycle race in Rome 1960.

Electrolytes

Our body fluids, like the contents of most living cells, consist of water, mineral salts and other dissolved substances. If sweat was made of water only, the concentration of salts in the body fluids would increase steadily and result in cellular poisoning just as in our example of the fish tank. This is avoided because sweat contains electrolytes in approximately the same concentration as they occur in the body. So it makes sense to replace essential electrolytes lost in sweat when 'quenching thirst' after or during exercise by drinking fruit or vegetable juices or specially developed 'sports' drinks.

Only fluid lost from the lungs is pure water and the amount may be greatly increased by overbreathing, but water lost by urine, faeces, sweat and evaporation is associated with the loss of electrolytes (see chapter 7). Electrolytes are involved in most biological processes and are of great importance in maintaining the osmotic balance of the body fluids and the acid-base equilibrium of the blood. Severe losses of fluid from the gut caused by vomiting or diarrhoea can incur heavy losses of water and electrolytes in a very short period of time, with serious consequences.

The fluid composition of the body is very complex and must be maintained within very exacting limits. This is done by osmosis.

When a solution of, for example, sugar is separated from pure water by a membrane which is permeable to water but not to sugar (a semipermeable membrane) water passes across the membrane into the sugar solution. This movement of water is called osmosis. If an external pressure is applied to the sugar solution the movement of water will be opposed. The pressure required to stop the movement completely is called the 'osmotic pressure' of the sugar solution. This osmotic pressure is greater the more concentrated the solution. Water will pass by osmosis from any solution having a weaker osmotic pressure to any having a stronger one, provided they are separated by a semipermeable membrane, until the two solutions have attained equal osmotic pressures. Walls of living cells are semipermeable membranes and much of the activity of the cells depends on osmosis.

It is beyond the scope of this book to go into a detailed description of all the physiological processes performed by the body to maintain its electrolyte concentration. Suffice to say that a considerable amount of the regulation occurs in the kidneys and is under hormonal control.

Of the minerals lost in sweat, sodium (Na^+) and chloride (Cl^-) are by far the most abundant. In the physiology of body fluids Na^+ and Cl^- are the ions mainly responsible for maintaining the water content of the extracellular space (ie interstitial and plasma water). This is done by keeping a constant relationship between the number of ions and water molecules. For example, if a great quantity of Na^+ and Cl^- ions were lost in sweat, the body could lose part of its control of the distribution and volume of extracellular water. If ions are lost, attempts are made to redistribute water in an effort to maintain the original water–ion relationship. Over time a severe sodium chloride depletion would lead to progressive water loss from the extracellular compartment of the body and, therefore, from the plasma volume. As we have said, a decrease in plasma volume can produce circulatory failure.

Although the body can adjust remarkably well to reduced intakes of sodium chloride by reducing the amount lost in sweat and urine, it is still necessary to replace electrolytes during periods of heavy sweating.

In one study it was observed that a 5 to 8 per cent reduction in body weight and a loss of 4.11 litres of sweat produced deficits in body Na^+ and Cl^- of about 5 to 7 per cent. At the same time total body potassium and magnesium, the two ions principally confined to the intracellular space, decreased less than 1.2 per cent. This work demonstrates that during prolonged exercise the only ionic deficits of any consequence are those of the extracellular fluid, ie Na^+ and Cl^-.

There is a greater requirement to replace body water than to replace electrolytes, though the latter are still important. As already mentioned, sports drinks are a good way of ensuring sufficient fluid replacement with the correct balance of electrolytes. However, commercial preparations can vary widely in composition, and their use has to be controlled wisely.

There are a number of points to consider when using sports drinks. Taking each of these in turn:

The temperature of the drink is important. Cold drinks between 4 °C and 10 °C (40 °F to 50 °F empty from the stomach faster than warm drinks and pass into the intestines quicker where they are absorbed into the body. Cold drinks can also provide a momentary temperature sink for body heat.

The greater the volume ingested (up to about 600 ml or just over 1 pint), the quicker the rate of emptying from the stomach. Moderate portions of 150 to 200 ml (approximately one-quarter to one-third of a pint) should be consumed every 15 minutes, though most athletes find this inconvenient and quickly incur a water imbalance.

As the intensity of exercise increases, the rate of emptying slows down, causing an increase in the danger of gastric upset. Prolonged work at a comfortable intensity (about 65 to 70 per cent of maximum) gives a constant rate of emptying.

The drink's concentration, and particularly its sugar content, also affects the rate of gastric emptying. The whole drink should remain hypotonic (ie a lower concentration in the drink than in the body fluids) with an osmolality around 200/litre. This is equivalent to a solution containing 2.5 per cent glucose.

The best advice during strenuous exercise is to drink before feeling thirsty and keep on drinking small volumes at frequent intervals. Replacement of fluids is essential and replacement of electrolytes is beneficial, particularly when undertaking long periods of exercise in warm conditions.

9 Body weight and composition

In many sports the participants' weight has a direct relevance to their ability to participate or excel. In boxing, wrestling or horse racing the fighters and jockeys need to maintain their weight within a narrow closely defined range. If it falls outside this range they are either penalised or not allowed to compete.

In other sports there are ideal weights in relation to body size, and athletes have to try and maintain them.

Body fat

A number of scientific studies have shown a high negative relationship between performance in various activities and the relative amount of body fat. In most sports it has been found that people with the higher percentage of body fat have the poorer performances. This is particularly true in sports where the body has to be propelled either vertically or horizontally through space, for example sprinting, high jumping or long jumping.

There have been some misconceptions that the bigger an athlete is the better the performance. This is only true where the increase in size is a true increase in lean weight (muscle) and not due to a deposition of fat. With the possible exception of the Japanese Sumo wrestler, the addition of fat just to increase body weight is detrimental to performance.

One of the problems in sport is assessing a person's ideal weight. Standard tables have been drawn up which are based on sex, height, build and weight, but unfortunately these are developed from data based on the population as a whole, and many athletes, as a consequence of training and selection, may have a heavy bone structure and large muscle mass. The problems occur when an athlete is 'overfat' rather than 'overweight' when compared against standard tables.

So body composition is more important than body weight and when considering body composition, the total body weight is considered in two parts: the lean weight and the fat weight.

Lean body weight is the part of the total body weight remaining after all body fat is removed. It is composed of muscle, skin, bone, organs and all other non-fat tissue. The fat weight is the estimated weight of the total body fat.

When working with body composition data these relationships are important:

total body weight = lean body weight + fat weight

relative body fat = (fat weight/total body weight) × 100

A number of methods have been developed to measure body composition. A common technique is densitometry which relies on underwater weighing. Subjects are weighed while totally submerged and after all air has been exhaled from their lungs. This weight is then corrected for the buoyancy effect of additional air trapped in the lungs and for gas in the intestinal tract. The weight and volume of the body is determined and from

47

these values the density can be calculated since

$$\text{density} = \frac{\text{mass}}{\text{volume}}$$

Information based on anatomical studies and work on cadavers has enabled factors to be determined for the density of lean tissue and body fat. This means that equations can be established which allow the estimation of relative body fat, and from this information a person's lean body weight and fat weight can be calculated.

Although this technique has its limitations, it does allow comparisons of body composition to be made. Other methods of estimating body composition include anthropometric measurements and skinfold fat thicknesses.

From the data obtained by the various methods it has been found that body composition values vary with the type of sport.

Sports with a high endurance component or a strict weight classification system will typically have athletes characterised by low relative body fat. For example, long-distance runners generally have less than 10 per cent body fat, whereas males and females in their late teens will average 13 to 16 and 22 to 25 per cent respectively. The female athlete is typically fatter than the male due to the sex-specific fat on breasts and hips.

Examples of body compositions of male and female athletes in selected sports are given in table 16.

Any serious assessment of an athlete's ideal weight should begin by determining body composition. If the percentage of fat is considerably higher than the range normally associated with the sport, a controlled programme of weight loss through diet and exercise should be undertaken. This programme should aim at losing about 1 kg (2 lb) per week. If any major change takes place in the athlete's weight the composition should be redetermined.

Any special diet for weight loss must be carefully evaluated before starting. Effective weight loss can only be achieved by reducing calorie intake to a point where intake is lower than expenditure. Since body fat contains some water it is not pure fat and has a calorie content of about 3500 calories per pound. So the loss of each pound of fat requires a deficit of energy expenditure over consumption of 3500 calories.

To lose 1 kg (2 lb) of fat a week, a person must reduce food consumption or increase energy expenditure by 1000 calories a day. This requires a major change in either food intake or exercise levels. Athletes in particular should only attempt to lose weight on soundly based, scientifically designed programmes. Many fad and crash diets make claims for enormous weight losses over short periods of time. Some of these can be dangerous with lasting effects. If the carbohydrate levels recommended in the diet are insufficient, the body will begin to break down its own proteins in muscle and organ tissue and enzymes. A major risk when this happens is that protein will be removed from heart muscle leaving the heart permanently weakened.

Another problem connected with the imbalance of nutrients in crash diets is if fat gets broken down at a faster rate than the body can use it, it may not be completely burned up. The result is the formation of ketone bodies and a condition known as

Table 16   *Body composition values*

Sport	Male Age	Relative fat (%)
canoeing	23.7	12.4
gymnastics	20.3	4.6
ice hockey	22.5	13.0
rowing	23.0	11.0
football	26.0	9.6
swimming	21.8	8.5
shot put	22.0	19.6
Female		
basketball	19.1	20.8
gymnastics	20.1	15.5
	23.0	11.0
skiing (Alpine)	19.5	20.6
swimming	19.4	26.3
running (distance)	19.9	19.2
jumping/hurdling	20.3	20.7
pentathlon	21.5	11.0

(Data from Wilmore 1982)

ketosis. Ketone bodies is the name given to the penultimate products of fatty acid metabolism (acetoacetic acid, betahydroxybutyric acid and acetone). They can be oxidised only at a limited rate and when their production is excessive they accumulate in the blood and are excreted in the urine. In ketosis, water loss can occur from the body's efforts to excrete ketone bodies through the urinary tract. This water loss is often perceived as weight loss. The presence of ketone bodies at high levels in the body can lead among other things to kidney and bladder damage.

Dieting

Athletes should avoid crash diets unless they are under medical supervision. Calorie intake should not be less than 800 calories per day during a day in which training does not take place, and if the normal calorie intake is in excess of 3000 calories per day the diet should aim to reduce this intake by between 1000 and 1200 calories a day.

The first week of a diet will show a deceptively rapid loss of weight, often as high as 2.25 kg (5 lb). This is not fat loss but the loss of water from glycogen. As the glycogen stores are used up, water is eliminated giving what appears to be a rapid weight loss. This water is replaced after a few days and the weight loss seen in subsequent weeks is mainly from fat.

It is very important that a person on a calorie-reduced diet compensates for the reduced intake of non-energy related nutrients, the vitamins, minerals and fibre. It is advisable to take a good multivitamin and multimineral supplement to ensure the requirements are maintained. Extra fibre should also be eaten. Fibre does not contribute calories to the diet but can add significantly to the bulk of a calorie-reduced diet, and so help offset the problem of constipation which often happens during dieting.

Participants in sports where body weight is part of the selection criteria (eg horse racing, boxing and wrestling) may attempt to lose weight for a brief period by restricting water as well as food intake. Studies indicate that this technique will markedly decrease muscular endurance, tissue glycogen levels and muscle water content. It can also lead to impairment of the normal functioning of the body's temperature regulation system. Work with American college wrestlers has shown that they entered competitions in a state of dehydration as a result of attempts to invoke rapid weight loss. It was also found that a wrestler in the 150 lb (70 kg) weight class could lose between 1.3 and 2.3 kg of fluid per hour during strenuous exercise or competitions in a hot environment. If this water loss is not replenished, the effects of dehydration can lead to exhaustion or heat stroke. Participants in weight-controlled sports must be educated on the need to replace fluids and the importance of competing in a hydrated state.

10 The teenage athlete

Younger athletes, particularly teenagers, need to known the importance of good nutrition as adolescence produces so many dramatic physical changes.

Growth rate increases rapidly around the onset of puberty and maintains this high rate of growth for two to three years. In girls the most rapid changes normally take place between 11 and 14 years, and in boys it is usually a little later at between 13 and 16 years. But there is a wide individual variation with some teenagers developing either much earlier or much later than the average.

Nutrient requirements

Many levels of nutrients required by growing teenagers are considerably higher in proportion to body size and weight than they will be in adult years. For example, the United Kingdom recommended daily amount of calcium for both boys and girls between 9 and 14 years of age is 700 mg per day compared with the RDA of 500 mg per day for adults. Similarly the nicotinic acid requirements for mid teenagers are also higher than for adults.

Evidence from dietary surveys carried out in the United Kingdom shows that teenagers' eating habits leave a lot to be desired. There is a tendency to skip breakfast and to reduce calorie intake, and the results of one survey showed that as many as 25 per cent of a sample of mid teenagers did not normally have breakfast (table 17). The same survey also showed that 8 per cent of the sample (one in twelve of the children) only had one proper meal a day.

The United Kingdom RDA for energy for the 15 to 17-year-olds is 2880 kcal for boys and 2150 for girls. Sports training could increase these needs and the high calorie requirements are unlikely to be met if meals are habitually missed.

Teenage athletes need to maintain higher-than-average intakes of iron. During the period of rapid growth the body's blood supplies and iron reserves expand and the extra iron is necessary to maintain normal haemoglobin levels and to build iron reserves. The onset of menstruation in girls produces additional demands on iron levels, and the serious teenage athlete undergoing strenuous training may also be susceptible to sports anaemia. A positive effort must be made to ensure that the diet contains foods rich in iron (chapter 7, table 11) and that vitamin C intake is increased to aid the absorption of non-haem iron.

Calcium intake during puberty is also very important as the body is laying down a large quantity of additional bone mass. In the USA the calcium intake is regarded as being so critical that the RDAs for calcium for both boys and girls in the 13 to 18-year age group are 1200 mg per day, over 60 per cent more than those recommended in the United Kingdom.

There is a strong possiblity that teenage athletes of both sexes may need to take some form of mineral supplementation, particularly during periods of heavy training.

Table 17   *Proportion of children eating breakfast in three different age groups*

	5–10 years (%)	10–14 years (%)	14–18 years (%)
cooked	6	10	9
cereal-based	67	52	47
bread-based	15	19	20
snack	4	6	5
nothing	8	13	20

(National Dairy Council Report 1982)

Body-building

Many teenage male athletes have a desire to increase their strength, muscle mass and body weight. Contrary to popular myth, there is no specific nutrient, hormone, drug or protein compound that will increase muscle mass. The only way muscles can be developed is by undertaking a planned course of training over a number of months. During this training it will be necessary to increase the total daily calorie intake by up to 1000 calories a day, and this may require a complete restructuring of the diet. An increased food energy intake, combined with a well-designed weight-training programme, should stimulate an increase in muscle weight. A well-planned programme of diet and training can achieve a weight gain of about 0.5 kg (1 lb) per week in mid to late teenagers.

This rate may be regarded as being too slow by some who may be tempted to investigate drugs such as the androgenic hormones, so-called steroids. In healthy young men these drugs are ineffective in increasing either muscle mass or muscle strength and can be associated with serious toxic side effects. It is also unnecessary to consume disproportionate amounts of protein or amino acids as the excess is more likely to be converted to expensive energy rather than laid down as muscle.

It is important that any muscle-building or weight-gain programme is supervised to ensure that the body fat levels are not increasing. If this happens the calorie intake may have to be slightly reduced.

It is also important that young athletes and their coaches are aware of the need to assess the body's degree of maturation before embarking on intensive training programmes. Young men first grow in height and only after the rapid gains in height will they begin to show significant increases in weight due to increases in muscle size. This sequence is regulated and controlled by the normal hormonal changes directly related to sexual maturation that occur during adolescence. Most boys will not have the potential for increasing muscle mass or strength until approximately twelve to 18 months after their height gain has reached peak velocity. A rule-of-thumb measure of the male body's ability to increase muscle is the development and distribution of genital hair. It is only when hair has begun to develop on the inner aspects of the thigh that the body has reached the state of maturation which allows the muscles to develop. Training prior to this stage may improve the strength of the muscle but will only produce small changes in the amount of muscle.

Training in hot conditions

A young athlete who is prepubescent or in the early stages of puberty can have a fluid balance and thermoregulation problem which is often not appreciated by their coaches or people supervising them.

A prepubertal child's skin does not produce sweat as effectively as that of an adult and it does not have the ability to produce a more dilute and abundant sweat with repeated training in the heat. As a consequence the body of a prepubertal child is less efficient at thermoregulation than one that has passed through puberty and is less able to adapt to exercise under warm conditions. This can place the younger athlete at a greater risk of heat-induced collapse or heat stroke, and particular attention must be paid to maintaining adequate hydration. To compound the problem, it has been found that younger athletes are able to develop a sense of well-being more rapidly than older athletes when exercising in the heat. This psychological adjustment to the warm environment is not met by a complete physiological adjustment and this increases the risk of heat-induced problems.

Education

During adolescence the body's demand for nutrients is at one of its peaks and ironically it is also often the time when poor eating habits are at their worst. The relaxation of parental control on meals, an obsession with weight particularly amongst girls, and changes in lifestyle all combine to have a detrimental impact on the teenager's nutrient intake. In addition, nutrition education in schools is still sparse and information from television and magazines is often conflicting.

It is therefore not surprising that very few teenagers are following even the most elementary nutritional guidelines in their diet and it is even more important that the aspiring teenage athlete is encouraged to eat wisely.

11 The diabetic athlete

Many diabetics, at some time or other, are faced with the dilemma of whether or not it is safe for them to take up a sporting activity or indeed continue with their already chosen sport. It can be a very traumatic experience when you discover you are suffering from diabetes. There is so much to do in adjusting to a new lifestyle it is understandable that many fears still remain and that the full consequences and tolerances of the disease may not at first be totally appreciated. But it is important, especially for the young diabetic, to keep fit and active to maintain a healthy circulation.

This chapter explains this condition and gives constructive advice to both the diabetic athlete and the coach on how best to approach physical exercise.

Diabetes mellitus, to give the disease its full title, is a common complaint which affects about one in every 100 people. It is more commonly found in women than men and becomes more frequent with increasing age. The disease can affect children but only about 5 per cent of all cases are in the age group 0–20 years.

Diabetes is a disease in which the body is unable to break down and utilise all the nutrients in the diet. Excessive amounts of sugar, instead of being burned up as energy, accumulate in the blood and spill over into the urine. Too much fat also builds up in the blood and some of the protein is converted to sugar instead of being used in its more usual role of producing muscles and replacing damaged tissues. Over a period of time this high blood glucose level can damage the eyes, kidneys and nerves as well as other parts of the body. All these problems are due to one basic cause: the diabetic's inability to produce enough insulin to utilise these foods properly.

Insulin

The hormone insulin is produced by the pancreas, a gland which lies close to the stomach (see fig 4). About 98 per cent of the gland is concerned with producing digestive enzymes which pass into the duodenum. Only the remaining 2 per cent of the pancreas makes insulin. The cells which are responsible for insulin production are scattered throughout the pancreas (more than one million of them) and collectively known as the islets of Langerhans (after Paul Langerhans who discovered them in 1869). If these islets fail to produce insulin, or make too little, then diabetes results. The rest of the pancreas is almost never affected and this suggests that whatever the cause of diabetes, it is very specific. *Diabetes mellitus* is actually a group of metabolic disorders having in common an actual or relative lack of insulin.

In most young diabetics the pancreatic islets failure is complete and so they must rely on insulin injections for the rest of their lives (insulin must be injected since if taken orally it would be destroyed by the digestive enzymes). In most older patients the pancreatic islet failure is not complete and the gland still retains some capacity for insulin production. These patients do not usually need insulin injections and can normally be treated by dietary regulation. Diabetics who require insulin for survival are termed Type 1 diabetics and those who are non-insulin dependent, Type 2 diabetics.

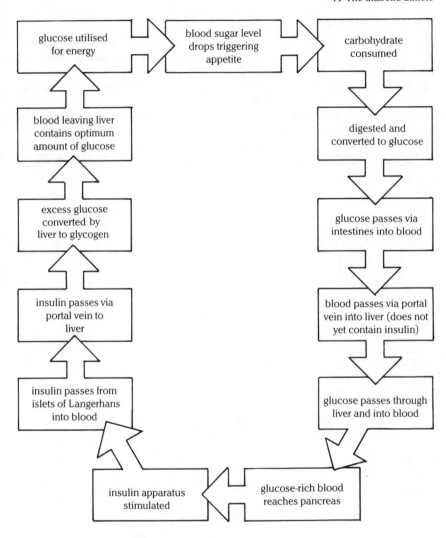

Fig 11   *Mechanism for glucose regulation in the body*

Once glucose enters the bloodstream, the body utilises as much as it needs for immediate energy. Any excess is stored in the liver either as triglyceride or glycogen and in the fat reserves as triglyceride. The whole process of glucose utilisation and storage is very complex and one of the most important factors in this operation is insulin (fig 11). While insulin is essential for breaking down glucose to energy, it is also required to prevent excessive fat breakdown and so it promotes energy storage.

55

Balancing blood sugar

In non-diabetics the blood sugar level is kept within fairly narrow limits and even after a large meal with considerable amounts of sugar it does not usually rise above 150 mg per 100 ml (8 mmol/litre). In non-diabetics enough insulin is produced by the pancreas to control blood sugar levels – rather like the thermostat on a central heating system.

Fig 12 illustrates that insulin levels in non-diabetics are highest when someone has just eaten and lowest when fasting. The relationship of insulin to other hormones ensures that the normal level of glucose in the blood remains relatively constant in most people, and regardless of whether a person fasts for a long period or eats a large meal, variations in blood glucose levels are minimal.

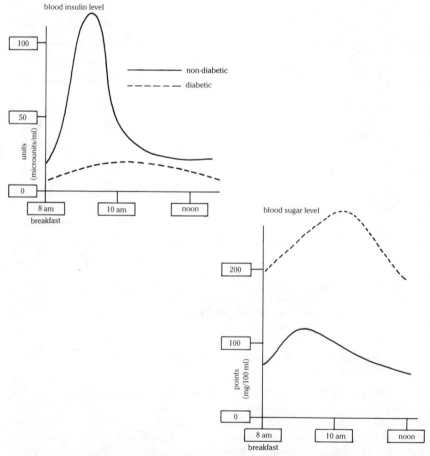

Fig 12   *Blood insulin and sugar levels in diabetics and non-diabetics*

If the body produces insufficient insulin to fully utilise or store all the glucose then glucose will accumulate in the blood and body tissues, especially after meals. Once the blood glucose level rises to about 180 mg/100 ml the kidneys are no longer able to hold the sugar back and it 'spills over' into the urine. The kidneys, which are large self-adjusting filters, have to work continuously to get rid of the excess sugar; this necessitates the use of large quantities of water resulting in dehydration and insatiable thirst.

The body needs energy to survive and since, in the diabetic, it cannot get all its requirements from dietary carbohydrate the body's protein and fat reserves are broken down as a source of energy (fig 13). This process which, incidentally, is the same as in starvation, is inefficient in terms of energy production.

Incomplete fat degradation results in the formation of acetone, or ketone bodies, which can be poisonous in large quantities. These ketone bodies are acidic and can cause nausea, vomiting, abdominal upsets, shortness of breath and confusion. As the diabetic becomes less able to cope with the rising ketone level the acid-base balance of the blood becomes disturbed. Also, the brain requires glucose for normal functioning and if the diabetic state becomes severe, the brain will suffer from lack of energy, and coma, followed by death, could result.

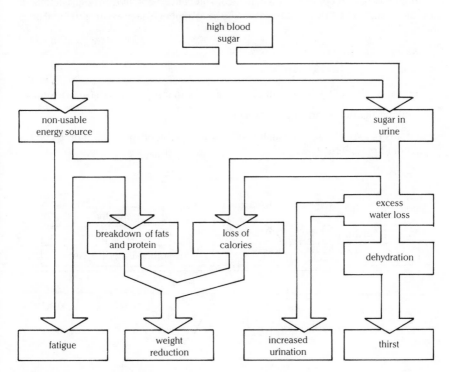

Fig 13 *Symptoms of diabetes*

Most diabetics develop the disease as adults, and many are overweight. Also, in the majority of these cases there is only a relative deficiency of insulin, ie the pancreas is still able to produce some insulin. It is vital that diabetics understand this since the degree of treatment of the disease is very much dependent upon their circumstances.

Complications

In recent years it has been discovered that another pancreatic hormone, glucagon, plays an important role in diabetes. Not only do diabetics have low insulin levels but they also exhibit a higher than normal level of glucagon which acts to suppress insulin thereby exacerbating the condition.

Blood circulation in diabetics can be seriously affected by the narrowing of the small blood vessels due to wall thickening. The main cause of this appears to be artery lining abnormalities, platelet malfunctions, and lipid–lipoprotein disturbances. These can lead to reduced sensation or numbness and because of this it is particularly important that athletes take special care of their feet. Any small cuts or cracked skin should be treated immediately before more serious problems develop. Shoes should be well-fitting to avoid blisters.

Another common complication which can affect the diabetic is hypoglycaemia, or low blood sugar (fig 14). This can be caused by a number of factors, the principal ones being

late or missed meals

accidental overdose of insulin

increased physical activity (without an increase in food or a decrease in insulin)

drinking alcohol on an empty stomach.

Symptoms of hypoglycaemia usually occur when the blood sugar level drops below 55 mg/dl (3 mmol/litre).

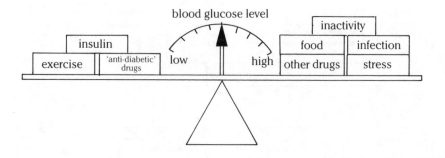

Fig 14   *Factors affecting blood glucose levels*

Although diabetic complications can be serious the course of diabetes in a person is very varied and it is difficult to predict which complications, if any, will occur. Careful monitoring and control of the condition at all times is the key to providing a lifestyle as trouble-free as possible, and at least if complications do arise they can be treated immediately.

Controlling diabetes

Physical activity is important for everybody but a long-term commitment to physical activity is a useful addition to diabetic control and may help prevent complications. Exercise can help to maintain blood sugar within normal levels, despite the fact that during prolonged mild-to-moderate exercise glucose utilisation may increase about 20-fold over the basal level and account for 25 to 40 per cent of the total oxidative fuel requirements. This is because for approximately the first 40 minutes of exercise the glucose pool is being replaced by an increased release of glucose from the liver.

Eventually, if the exercise continues for long enough, blood glucose levels will fall and there will be a progressive shift from carbohydrate to free fatty acid metabolism.

Once the activity has ceased, the depletion in muscle glycogen must be restored and a prolonged stimulation of glycogen synthetase (an enzyme which promotes glycogen synthesis) leads to an increase in glucose uptake. This replenishment of muscle and liver glycogen stores can take from 24 to 48 hours during which there is an improvement in glucose tolerance and diminished insulin requirement.

Recent studies have indicated that exercise increases cellular sensitivity to insulin in both diabetics and non-diabetics by significantly increasing the number of insulin receptors in proportion to the improvement in physical fitness.

A possible problem which Type 1 diabetics may face is what is called 'exercise-induced hypoglycaemia'. This risk can be reduced by decreasing the insulin dose, avoiding exercise during peak insulin effect, or taking a carbohydrate snack about half an hour prior to and during prolonged periods of activity. The use of non-exercised injection sites for insulin, eg the abdominal wall, could also help.

Further benefits that the diabetic can expect from regular exercise are weight reduction, better nutrient utilisation through improved muscle tone and strength, a reduction in lipid abnormalities, and a decrease in the high levels of plasma triglycerides coupled with an increase in the more beneficial high-density lipoproteins (HDL).

Diet is the most common method of diabetic treatment and more than one-third of all diabetics can be satisfactorily controlled solely by dietary manipulation. Reduction in total calories to achieve an ideal weight is also a prime objective of most diabetics.

However, methods of dietary control have been the subject of much concern and debate. It has often been suggested that diabetics should restrict the carbohydrate contribution in their diet, but more recent evidence seems to favour a diet high in complex carbohydrates. This results in greater carbohydrate tolerance and a reduced insulin requirement. Fibre-rich meals also reduce postprandial hyperglycaemia and glycosuria in Type 1 diabetics.

In general, dietary recommendations for the diabetic athlete are the same as those for the non-diabetic athlete and are summarised in table 18. The important points to

Table 18   *Dietary recommendations for the diabetic athlete*

If obese, reduce calories gradually until desired weight is achieved.

Increase intake of complex carbohydrates.

Reduce total fat, saturated fat, and cholesterol intakes.

Avoid simple sugars.

Eat well-balanced meals regularly.

---

be emphasised are

intake of simple sugars kept down to a minimum to avoid hyperglycaemic peaks

proper selection of foods to ensure adequate nutrition

total caloric intake sufficient to satisfy energy expenditure

proper timing of meals, especially for Type 1 diabetics.

Diabetics need have no special worries about taking part in sport provided they fully understand both the benefits and possible dangers. Insulin-dependent diabetics will have to be particularly cautious to prevent hypoglycaemia, and this will probably involve a carefully worked out exercise programme in consultation with a medical advisor.

Activities should stop at the first sign of hypolycaemia and glucose or some carbohydrate snack eaten. It is also wise not to exercise alone and to ensure those around you are aware of your condition. Fluid replacement both during and after exercise is important to avoid dehydration.

A diabetic should not indulge in strenuous exercise without first having a full medical examination and only after reasonable diabetic control is established. A warm-up and cool-down period should also be allowed for in the activity. Above all, do not overdo it.

With experience, most diabetics learn how to regulate their eating habits in relation to the amount of exercise to be undertaken, and diabetic control need not be compromised to enjoy a full sporting life.

12 Special techniques

For many years it has been known that during an endurance activity both carbohydrates and lipids contribute to energy metabolism. Also, the faction of energy provided by carbohydrates during prolonged exercise depends, among other things, on its intake both before and during the activity. For this reason many athletes have turned their attention to dietary controls in an effort to attain maximum performance. One such technique is carbohydrate loading.

Carbohydrate loading

This is a technique which relies on the theory that if the glycogen stores in muscles are depleted then the muscle will take in and store a higher amount of glycogen than usual and these increased stores will be available for utilisation during competition. This is done with a precisely structured regime of dieting and exercise for a prescribed period prior to the event. But before a more detailed discussion on this, some of the more important factors on which this theory is based will be re-emphasised.

When the glycogen stores in exercised muscles are exhausted, the muscles are unable to continue high-intensity activity, and although fats also serve as a critical fuel during long-duration activity, it is the glycogen in muscle and glucose in blood that are the primary sources of energy for most athletic events. The body's glycogen stores are often less than that required for optimal performance and it is important for athletes to try to maximise these stores and minimise the rate at which they are depleted. The body's glycogen reserves are mobilised much more easily if their level was high prior to exercise. Once the glycogen reserves are exhausted, fatigue occurs. For most types of exercise it is advantageous to start with a high level of glycogen reserve.

If high carbohydrate reserves are necessary for stamina and depletion leads to exhaustion, what happens if an athlete drinks a glucose solution prior to an event to build up energy reserves? Glucose is quickly absorbed into the body and produces an energy 'high'. But this is followed by an energy 'low' due to a control mechanism whereby the pancreas secretes insulin into the bloodstream to counteract the high glucose level (fig 15). If this secretion of insulin is followed by a period of exercise, the combination of the two can induce a rapid decrease in blood glucose concentration which will eventually result in hypoglycaemia (low blood sugar). This hypoglycaemia may lead to fatigue which could diminish athletic performance. The 'low' may be countered to some extent by ingesting protein at the same time as the glucose.

In contrast to glucose, it has been shown that fructose causes significantly lower elevations in blood glucose (fig 15), and therefore little or no rise in blood insulin levels. In addition to sparing muscle glycogen, fructose taken before exercise does not reduce plasma-free fatty acids to the same extent as glucose and therefore allows more fat utilisation during exercise.

In a study of an English professional football team, the players were encouraged to take a high-carbohydrate diet for 36 hours preceding their Saturday match with a reduction in training on the Friday and only very light exercises on the Saturday

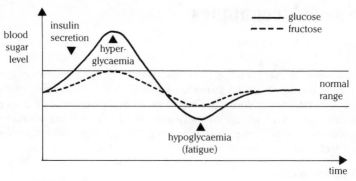

Fig 15   *Blood glucose level*   (From McCann 1980)

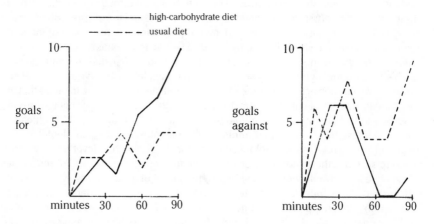

16a

	usual diet		high carbohydrate diet	
	first half	second half	first half	second half
goals for	8	10 (8)*	4	20 (15)
goals against	16	15 (12)	15	3 (1)

*Figure in brackets indicates goals in the final 30 minutes of match.

16b

Fig 16   *Comparison of a high-carbohydrate diet versus a normal diet on goals scored per 15-minute period (average of 20 matches)*   (From Muckle 1981)

morning. There was a significant improvement in their performance over a 20-match period as assessed by goals scored and goals conceded (fig 16a). The team's performance improved significantly and was especially noticeable in the final 30 minutes of the matches (fig 16b). Important points highlighted by this study were the fact that the players not on the high-carbohydrate diet had 20 to 50 per cent less ball contacts and involvement in play during the final 30 minutes of play, and the differences between the two groups of players was only significant in the second half of the game.

The aim of carbohydrate loading is to maximise glycogen stores in the muscles and liver because intense endurance activity depends on high levels of glycogen. The higher the glycogen reserves, the more fuel available to sustain endurance activity.

There is still considerable disagreement among experts regarding the beneficial effects of carbohydrate loading. In fact, some even say it is harmful.

Essentially the technique is a six-day programme. The first three days consist of heavy exercise to deplete the glycogen reserves in the muscles, coupled with a high-fat, high-protein diet which keeps the muscles deprived of glycogen (fig 17). During

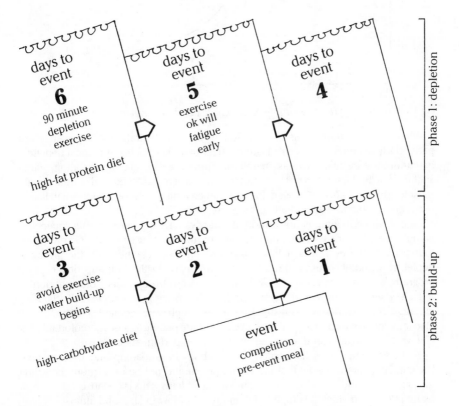

Fig 17   *Schedule for carbohydrate loading*

this exercise period it is necessary to use the muscles that will be used during the actual event, for example it is of no use to have a programme of swimming exercises if the event is to be a cycle race. This is to deplete the glycogen stores in the actual muscles where the extra stamina is required. After the initial three-day period, a high-carbohydrate diet should be consumed and training stopped. It is during this period that the muscles rebuild their glycogen reserves achieving a greater level than normal.

The high-carbohydrate diet should be based on such foods as pasta, cereals, potatoes and breads which consist of complex carbohydrates rather than simple sugars. This is because the complex starches are digested at a much slower rate and a hypoglycaemic response is avoided (fig 18).

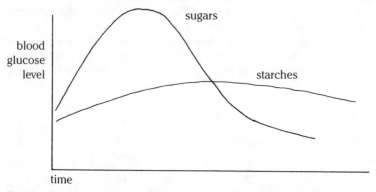

Fig 18 *Absorption rates of simple and complex carbohydrates*

When the programme is strictly followed, carbohydrate loading can work, particularly in endurance events lasting longer than 90 minutes. It is most beneficial in endurance events, such as marathon running or cross-country skiing, where stamina is a key factor. It is not suitable for events where, under normal conditions, the muscles do not drain of glycogen. In most trained athletes glycogen stores will last for between one and one-and-a-half hours of exercise.

Carbohydrate loading is not without its disadvantages. A serious consequence of carbohydrate loading is the disruption to the normal training schedule. On days six to four prior to the event the high-fat, high-protein diet, together with the glycogen-depleting workout, causes the athlete to tire easily. In the build-up phase of the programme it is necessary to cease training to ensure a 'super concentration' of muscle glycogen. These two factors can have immense pyschological effects. Also, although carbohydrate is easily digested, it has a high water content so extra water is also laid down in the muscles. This can cause some people to feel uncomfortable and stiff which could also produce an adverse effect on performance.

There are other risks associated with carbohydrate loading and the American Dietetic Association warns that the technique should not be used more than three times per year, and probably not at all by young athletes. This is because the diet is an extreme one and since it is high in fat and protein, low in fibre and almost certainly deficient in some vitamins and minerals, it would be dangerous if it was maintained over a long period. It can produce some physiological irregularities and therefore anybody suffering from diabetes, cardiovascular disease or high-serum triglycerides should only undertake the programme in consultation with their medical advisor.

Research has shown that diet plays a major role in optimising performance, and it is understandable that athletes will strive to increase their carbohydrate reserves in an attempt to improve stamina. But there are many considerations to be taken into account when trying to achieve a greater degree of stamina, and carbohydrate loading is probably not the only method that will work for some athletes. It has inherent hazards and should be used cautiously. If misused it can reduce performance.

The traditional method of carbohydrate loading as described has been directly compared to a dietary regime that allowed the subjects to eat a normal mixed diet, where 50 per cent of the calories were obtained from carbohydrates, in place of the three-day high-fat, high-protein diet. No significant differences were found between the two regimes, and the researchers concluded that a trained athlete can develop a very large muscle glycogen store simply by eating a carbohydrate-rich diet for the 72 to 48-hour period before the endurance event provided that no exercise is undertaken during this period. There is sufficient evidence to show that carbohydrate loading can increase an athlete's stamina. Whether this is reflected as an increase in performance still remains open to question.

Drugs and stimulants

The search for methods to rapidly increase stamina and performance has over the years encouraged many people to experiment with a variety of compounds. Unfortunately the 'magic' food ingredient still remains elusive and is found only in the fantasy world of cartoon characters such as Popeye and Desperate Dan. As a consequence many athletes have been tempted to experiment with drugs.

There are some components of food products such as caffeine, phenylalanine and octacosanol which have acquired a reputation as performance enhancers. Whether this reputation is justified is still open to conjecture.

Caffeine, naturally present in coffee, tea, cola drinks and chocolate, is taken by many athletes, particularly marathon runners, as a means of stimulating the body and increasing the capacity for muscular work. However, caffeine is a drug which acts as a stimulant and will, depending on the dosage, affect the body by raising the heartbeat and basal metabolic rate, promoting secretion of gastric acids and increasing the production of urine. Since it passes easily through biological membranes, caffeine is rapidly absorbed from the gastrointestinal tract and becomes widely distributed throughout the body. Studies have shown that caffeine promotes fat metabolism and slows down the rate of muscle glycogen usage leading to a greater endurance capacity. But it has also been noted that caffeine has a stimulating effect on the body's sympathetic nervous system, producing a lessening of the person's subjective estimate of the degree of effort. At least part of the performance advantage of caffeine is likely to be psychological.

The diuretic effect of caffeine cannot be overlooked and, as highlighted in chapter 8, water is an essential nutrient and dehydration must be avoided. Any agent which speeds up the dehydration process is counterproductive to the body's efficiency.

Some amino acids, in particular L-phenylalanine and tyrosine, are being used as alternatives to drugs as they are reputed to be ergogenic (increase performance) without the side effects associated with drugs such as amphetamines and steroids.

Research is showing little or no evidence of the efficacy of most of the amino acid supplements currently being recommended when the protein content of the diet is adequate, and there appears to be no justification for specific amino acid supplementation.

One of the more recent supplements used by athletes is octacosanol. This is a 28 carbon atom chain alcohol found principally in wheatgerm oil. There have been a number of studies on the effects of octacosanol and wheatgerm oil on physical fitness but at present there is no unequivocal evidence to support its use in sport. All studies to date indicate that intense physical training itself is essential to improvement of endurance, stamina and strength. In the studies where octacosanol may have been beneficial, the results of the training far outweigh the alleged effects of octacosanol.

A multitude of other compounds such as ginseng and bee pollen have also been credited with improvements in performance, and doubtless over the years there will be many more. Much of the evidence for these preparations is anecdotal or subjective and possibly contains an element of the 'placebo effect'.

Although in some cases there may be a basis for the claims it is only when controlled objective trials stand up to scientific scrutiny that reliance can be placed on them.

13 Theory into practice (i): meal planning

There is a popular misconception amongst many athletes and coaches in Britain that the only good way to build up for an event is to eat large quantities of red meat such as steak.

For many years sportsmen and women have been brought up to believe the myth that the way to success is built on the consumption of large quantities of protein, and interviews and surveys have shown that meat, particularly red meat, is seen as being the most important component of their diets.

Biasing the diet

If the optimum performance is to be achieved, this myth has to be exploded. Far more benefit can be obtained by biasing the diet in favour of carbohydrates, particularly the complex carbohydrates, for the week or so immediately before an event. This does not mean that meats should be excluded but they should be consumed in moderation and not form the major part of the diet. The choice of meat can also help. White chicken meat (breast) has a similar protein content to rump steak but contains only a third of the amount of fat. Pork should be avoided because of its very high fat content and lamb needs to be prepared so that most of the fat is removed before cooking. With the exception of duck and goose, most poultry and game birds provide a good source of protein with a low fat content. Another excellent source of meat protein with a low fat content is found in white fish. Fish should be grilled or steamed and not fried. Offal in the form of liver and kidney can provide a good source of protein and relatively high amounts of the vitamins B_2, B_{12}, folic acid, niacin and vitamin C.

Meat, with the exception of liver, contains no carbohydrate and liver normally contains less than 5 per cent carbohydrate.

Even with sports requiring considerable strength, the daily protein requirement is unlikely to be in excess of 20 per cent of the total calorie intake. So a person consuming 4000 calories would need 200 g of protein. The carbohydrate required in a 'strength' sport will be about 45 per cent of the total energy, which means that the 4000-calorie consumer will need 480 g of carbohydrate. The quantity of carbohydrate required is almost two-and-a-half times that of protein.

If you look through the food composition tables (appendix 2), you will see that no single food contains the proportions of the energy nutrients in anywhere near the recommended ratios. This means that to achieve the required intakes, a whole range of foods must be eaten each day.

The four food groups

To obtain a balance of all the nutrients, dietitians have looked at various ways of classifying foods. One method, developed in the USA, is based on the concept of the four basic food groups. This places foods into four groups based on origin to give

milk and dairy products group

meat and fish group

fruit and vegetable group

grain and cereal group.

The fruit and vegetable group is subdivided into

dark green or yellow vegetables

other vegetables

citrus fruits

other fruits.

This is to ensure maximum benefit from the vitamins. Dark green and yellow vegetables normally have a high beta-carotene (provitamin A) content, and citrus fruits are particularly rich in vitamin C.

So a daily diet can be planned by defining the amount of food required from each group. By doing this it is theoretically possible to obtain the full requirements of all the essential nutrients.

The milk and dairy products group supplies protein, fat, calcium, magnesium, vitamin A and other vitamins and minerals. The meat and fish also provide protein and fat and some vitamins and minerals.

The fruits and vegetables, although contributing carbohydrate, are also a rich source of dietary fibre and, in addition, many fruits and vegetables contain relatively high levels of vitamins.

The grain and cereal group has relatively high levels of carbohydrates and low levels of fat, and whole-grain products also contain dietary fibre.

By calculating the amount of food required from each group it is possible to develop a range of daily menus which will deliver the desired quantities of nutrients, yet allow some flexibility for personal choice.

This technique is the one used by dietitians when designing special diets for medical purposes, and an example of how this can be applied to the development of guidelines for a balanced diet for athletes is given in table 19.

Table 19   *Balanced diet for athletes: general guidelines*

	3000 kcal/day *(12 550 kJ)*	*4000 kcal/day* *(16 736 kJ)*	*5000 kcal/day* *(20 920 kJ)*
Cereal group cereals, grains, bread, pasta, rice	14 servings	19 servings	26 servings
Fruit/vegetable group fresh, frozen, canned, dried or juice	14 servings	16 servings	18 servings
Dairy foods group milk, cheese, yoghurt, ice cream (preferably low fat, eg skimmed milk)	1 litre or equivalent	1.5 litres or equivalent	2 litres or equivalent
Meat group lean meat, poultry, fish, seafood	250 g	300 g	350 g
Fats/oils group butter, margarine, cooking oil	10 teaspoons	12 teaspoons	15 teaspoons

Explanation of servings

Cereal group

1 serving
    = 1 slice bread
    = ½ large roll
    = 1 crumpet
    = ⅓ cup (28 g, 1 oz) rice or pasta
    = 1 cup (28 g, 1 oz) ready-to-eat cereal
    = ½ cup (28 g, 1 oz) cooked cereal or muesli

Fruit/vegetable group

1 serving
    = ½ to 1 cup cooked or raw fruit or vegetables
    = 1 piece of fruit
    = 150 ml fruit juice

Daily requirement should include servings from
                dark green, orange vegetables
                other vegetables
                citrus fruits
                other fruits

Dairy foods group

300 ml skimmed milk	= 200 g low-fat yoghurt
	= 1 scoop ice cream
	= 150 g cottage cheese

Using good diet to the full

How can a coach or individual modify a diet to optimise the advantages of good nutrition? First, it is important to have a good understanding of the composition of the athlete's existing diet. People have their individual food fads and fancies and it is more realistic to make modifications and adjustments to a diet with which a person is familiar than to try and convert to a completely alien menu.

Full information on the existing diet is essential for making good nutrition part of the training process. Once a person has learnt to check and understand their own dietary habits, they will find it very much easier to make the modifications.

Keeping an accurate daily food diary (fig 19) is the key to becoming aware of what is actually being eaten. Ideally the diary should be kept for a seven-day period as this usually picks up most normal variations in dietary habits. If the seven days are not feasible a diary conscientiously maintained over at least three days, preferably but not

Date: 21/9/85   Day of diet: *Saturday 21st.*   Day: 1

Meal period	Time of day	Place	Food description	Weight (g)	Waste (g)	Drink	Amount	Actual weight	Code*
Breakfast	8·15	Home	Corn flakes (Tesco)	31	—	Tea with milk	2 cups	31	48
			Milk – whole	85	—			85	124
			Raisins	15	—			15	809
			Toast - 2 slices wholemeal	56	—			56	30
			Margarine about	6	—			6	187
			marmalade · homemade	13	—			13	853
Snack	10.30	Gym	Mars bar	42	—	diluted orange squash (Robinsons)	1 plastic cup	42	861
								about 10	884
Lunch	1·15	Home	Tomato soup (Heinz can)	225	—	Water	1 plastic cup	225	950
			Sandwich						
			4 slices wholemeal bread	131	—	Water	1 glass		
			Butter	14	—			131	30
			Corned beef (from can)	96	-	Coffee with milk	1 cup	14	140
			lettuce	7	—			96	393
			Apple (Cox?)	138	16			7	606
								122	675

Fig 19   *Food diary*

*Code refers to
food item reference in
Paul and Southgate (1978).

necessarily consecutive, will supply a large amount of valuable information on eating habits, size of meals, and times of eating and drinking in relation to exercise periods.

When keeping the food diary write down absolutely everything that is consumed as both food and drink during the 24-hour period. This includes all snacks, alcoholic beverages, sweets and even drinks of water. The estimates of portion sizes should be as accurate as the circumstances allow. It is not practical to weigh portions of food when eating out for example, and the measures may have to be related to the number of serving spoons, cups, or some other estimate.

Whenever possible the actual weight of each serving or component of the meal should be recorded. The best way to do this is to use a small 'add-on' type of kitchen scale. This is the type that can be adjusted to zero between each weighing. To weigh a meal using this method the plate is first placed on the scale and the pointer adjusted to zero. The first serving is added and the weight recorded. The scale is then reset to zero and the second item added. This can be repeated until all the servings of the course have been added to the plate.

All waste must be weighed and recorded after the meal. This will include bones and skin from meat or fish, uneaten portions, residues on the plate (gravy or sauces) and fruit stones and cores. This weight should be deducted from the initial weight of the food item. For example:

apple 86 g – waste (core) 17 g = actual consumption 69 g

When certain food items are used continually throughout the day (eg milk, coffee powder, fruit squash) it is often more convenient to remove the items from a pre-weighed container and record the cumulative usage at the end of the day. When doing this ensure that only one person uses the container and that its weights are recorded at the start and end of each day, the difference between the two weights being the daily usage.

The labels on cans or packets of food products often help in determining a portion size as the weight of the total contents has to be shown on the label, and many manufacturers are now also giving additional nutritional information.

The diary should include as much detail as possible about the food. For example, all components of a mixed salad should be listed, together with the amount and type of any salad dressing. The amount of margarine or butter added to a baked potato should be noted as should the sugar added to coffee or tea.

The time and place where the food was consumed should also be recorded. This is of particular importance when the food is consumed away from the normal eating place.

The easiest way to keep the diary accurately is to carry a small pocket notebook and pencil and record each intake immediately after consumption. This information can later be transferred to the diary sheet.

Selection of meals during the diary days must not be biased by the person's desire to please. There is a great temptation to alter selection and intake to 'improve' what they may consider to be weaknesses in their dietary habits.

When the diary is completed it will immediately begin to reveal information such as the relationship of meal and snack times to training and exercise periods, the type of food preferred for each meal, and the amount of liquid taken in during the day. It can also be seen whether the food is being obtained from all four food groups.

A more detailed study of the diary will give the quantity of food and drink consumed, an estimate of the total energy content, the ratios of the energy nutrients, and an indication of the amounts of minerals and vitamins which are likely to have been consumed during the day.

To obtain this nutritional information use food composition tables which give the details of the nutrient content of virtually all foods. These tables can normally be found in good reference libraries. They are also used regularly by dietitians, and it is most useful to get a dietitian's help and advice before undertaking a detailed analysis of the diet.

By using these tables anyone can get an indication of the structure of their diet in terms of the ratio of energy nutrients and total energy contribution.

It is also important at this stage to check that the diet contains foods from all four groups, that there is a sufficient contribution from milk or yoghurt and that all the vegetable and fruit subgroups are represented.

Once the total energy intake for each day is known, it should be checked to see if it is valid for the individual. To do this is somewhat tedious but necessary, and requires that the athlete maintains a weight chart over a period of weeks. It is important that the weight is measured under exactly the same conditions each day, and the recommended time is first thing in the morning after going to the toilet and before any food or drink is consumed. If the chart shows that the weight has remained almost constant over the period, the energy intake is about right. If the weight shows a slow increase it means that the energy intake is slightly higher than expenditure through exercise, and the level of food consumption may need to be reduced. On the other hand, a slow decrease in weight indicates that expenditure is exceeding intake.

Assuming that the individual is maintaining an acceptable weight, the next stage is to determine the proportions of each of the energy nutrients contributing to the total energy, not forgetting any alcohol which may have been consumed. The contribution of each of these nutrients must then be calculated in terms of the percentage of the total energy, for example:

$$\frac{\text{energy contribution from all fat sources (kcal or kJ)}}{\text{total energy (kcal or kJ)}} \times 100$$

In most unmodified British diets we would expect to see about 40 to 42 per cent of the diet as fat, 13 to 15 per cent as protein and 43 to 47 per cent as carbohydrate.

The next stage, which may require the help of a professional dietitian, is to look at ways of modifying the diet to give the preferred ratios of 50 per cent carbohydrate, 35 per cent fat and 15 per cent protein. The sources of fat in the current diet must first be identified. These will come mainly from the meat and dairy products but also from confectionery, cakes and biscuits. About half the calories in most sweet biscuits come from fats.

Dietary changes

The typical changes one should be looking for to improve the diet are a reduction in the fat levels by about one-sixth (16 per cent), an increase in the carbohydrate levels by about one-eighth (12 per cent), and an increase in protein by about one-seventh to one-sixth (14 to 16 per cent).

The reduction of fat should be taken from the animal fats, the fats associated with meat, and dairy fats. A significant reduction can be made by grilling rather than frying meat and fish, using skimmed or low-fat milk, avoiding fried foods such as potato chips and potato crisps. All visible fat should be trimmed off meat before cooking.

The calorie content of the fat which has been removed should be replaced with foods high in complex carbohydrates (starchy foods) such as breads, cereals, rice, pasta and boiled or baked potatoes. These foods are all good for building glycogen stores.

Some of these changes can be made relatively easily. For example, substituting porridge or breakfast cereal and toast for a fried breakfast of bacon, egg and fried bread, or choosing an Italian pasta dish such as spaghetti instead of steak in a restaurant (training often requires sacrifices!).

Recent research is showing that the simple carbohydrates found in fruits and the sugar in sweets, chocolates, soft drinks and biscuits do not build the glycogen stores as well as the complex carbohydrates. In addition, sweets, chocolate bars, biscuits and soft drinks are normally poor in important micronutrients and because of this most confectionery products are often referred to as supplying 'empty calories', ie the only nutritional contribution is energy. A high consumption of simple carbohydrates may also cause blood lipid levels to increase.

In summary, the main dietary changes needed are reduction of the fat content with emphasis on animal fats, a reduction in sugar and other simple carbohydrates and replacement of the energy contributed by these two categories by adding complex carbohydrates in the form of starchy foods. These changes alone can have a significant effect on the glycogen status and endurance of the body.

Proteins

Analysing the diet will also indicate the level and sources of protein. Normally only minor increases to protein intake will be required. Good animal sources of protein which do not have a high fat content are chicken and turkey, grilled liver, grilled or poached white fish, cottage cheese, skimmed milk and low-fat yoghurts. Vegetable protein can be obtained from low-fat soya flour, soya protein isolates, soya products such as tofu, haricot beans, butter beans and lentils. Cereal products such as wheat bran, wholemeal flour, oatmeal and macaroni contain both protein and complex carbohydrates.

Many vegetable proteins have a lower content of some essential amino acids (particularly methionine) which can result in a lower nutritive value. But this is only of concern in a strict vegetarian diet where there is no intake of animal proteins to supply the limiting amino acids.

Many athletes, particularly those in sports requiring strength, like to supplement their diet with proprietary high-protein drinks. The advantage of these is that they can contribute accurate quantities of protein without the fat which normally accompanies meat protein. Where these preparations are based entirely on vegetable protein ensure that the product is fortified with the essential amino acids to improve its nutritive value. For example, isolated soya protein powder, which is often used in supplements, has a protein efficiency ratio (PER) of between 1.8 and 1.9. When fortified with additional methionine the PER increases to 2.5, or to the same value as casein (milk protein).

If the diet contains about 15 per cent of its energy value as protein from a variety of animal and vegetable sources it is unlikely that an athlete will benefit from the consumption of high levels of single amino acid supplements which have recently become popular. Remember, when the body's protein intake greatly exceeds its requirements, the excess protein can be converted to energy. The excessive consumption of protein can be an expensive way of obtaining energy.

Fibre

Once the energy nutrient levels in the diet have been adjusted, the next nutrient to consider is fibre. Investigations into dietary intakes in the United Kingdom show that the fibre content of the typical daily diet is between 15 and 20 g. Most authorities now agree that this should be increased to between 30 and 35 g per day. High levels of dietary fibre are found in wheat bran, wholemeal flour, soya flour, haricot beans, peas, apricots, blackcurrants, figs and prunes. Almost all fruits and vegetables contain some dietary fibre.

To obtain the recommended levels of fibre, wholemeal bread should replace white bread. Bran-fortified breakfast cereals are an excellent source, and wholewheat versions of macaroni and other pastas are also now available in shops. The fibre content of most foods can be found in the food composition tables.

Minerals and vitamins

The diet should also be checked for the two minerals calcium and iron. Athletes need sufficient quantities of both these minerals each day. The higher-than-normal protein consumption associated with the high-calorie diet can lead to calcium excretion and this calcium must be replaced. Athletes, particularly women, on daily energy consumptions over 4000 calories should aim to take in between 1200 and 1500 mg calcium per day. Although this can be achieved by selecting foods particularly high in calcium (see table 10, page 34), it may be necessary to add the insurance of a calcium supplement. Similarly, higher-than-average intakes of iron are needed. The preferred source of iron is animal or haem iron found in liver, kidneys, black pudding and meat (table 11, page 36). As with calcium it may be worth considering modest iron supplementation as dietary surveys in the United Kingdom have shown that many people have difficulty obtaining their full requirements from their diet. The consumption of foods high in vitamin C will help the absorption of iron from the diet.

The help of a qualified dietitian may be necessary for calculating the vitamins and trace minerals in the diet as vitamins particularly can be lost or destroyed during food preparation. Work on the vitamin content of food served in catering establishments has shown that peas and cabbage kept in warm serving containers for 20 minutes will have lost more than one-third of their vitamin C content. As the athlete's needs of some vitamins, particularly the energy-related B vitamins, are higher than average, the daily consumption of a modest multivitamin multimineral supplement is worth considering.

Fluids

The food diary should also record fluid consumption and no diet for athletes is complete unless the daily liquid losses are compensated by intake. Adequate fluid intakes must be built into both the diet and the training programme to ensure that the body remains in a constant state of hydration.

As the sensations of thirst are normally triggered after about 0.5 to 1 per cent of the body weight of liquid has been lost (ie a loss of between 375 cl and 750 ml in a 75 kg person), the replacement liquid to quench thirst is often of insufficient volume to balance the loss. To maintain the body in a hydrated state drink more fluid than is dictated by thirst. The constant replacement of liquid during training and participation must become part of the athlete's self-discipline.

There is a relatively simple technique for estimating the amount of liquid each day. This is done by recording body weight immediately before and immediately after each training session. The difference between the two weights is all water loss.

There is no direct relationship between the amount of sweat felt on the body and the actual weight loss, as the humidity of the air will affect the rate at which sweat evaporates from the skin.

Keep records for at least a week and calculate the average value for the losses by adding all the daily losses together and dividing by the number of days.

This average value can be used to calculate the percentage of body weight lost as fluid during training by using the formula

$$\text{percent fluid loss} = \frac{\text{average daily loss (kg or lb)}}{\text{normal body weight (kg or lb)}} \times 100$$

The greater the percentage body weight loss the more concerned one should be with ensuring adequate replacement.

Once the amount of fluid that needs replacing during exercise or training has been calculated, a programme of fluid intake must be worked out. If the body is hydrated at the beginning of the training session and the session is not very intense, resulting in a weight loss of less than 2 per cent, it is sufficient to drink the replacement liquids over a period of a few hours after the session. Drink more than is required to quench the thirst. It will take a considerable time for the water to get back to the cells and normal weight is only regained between 15 and 20 hours after training.

If a person sweats heavily or undertakes a very intense training session, it may be necessary to take in liquids during training. To do this, water or a 'sports drink' should be taken in small amounts of about half a glass (100 ml) at a temperature of about 15 °C (60 °F) at intervals of about 10 or 15 minutes. This prevents the stomach from getting too full and creating problems during training. It is important that the rest of the losses are made up after the training session.

Serious athletes should be particularly sensitive to their fluid needs and should develop a pattern of drinking which suits their own requirements.

When building up or replacing fluid levels drink water, fruit juices or squashes, non-carbonated soft drinks or proprietary sports drinks. Avoid tea, coffee or soft drinks containing caffeine because caffeine has a diuretic effect which makes the body discharge liquid at a greater rate than normal. Carbonated drinks should also be avoided immediately before and during training or sports events.

14 Theory into practice (ii): selection of meals

The wide variation in personal preferences, eating habits and intakes means it is almost impossible to prescribe the universal diet, and it is also not within the scope of this book to provide an exhaustive list of recipes.

But it is possible to give examples of the type of selection which should be made at meal times and to give guidance on dishes which should be selected or avoided.

You will already have appreciated that with a little care good nutrition can still be achieved in our present society where nearly half the meals are eaten away from the home in schools, works canteens, restaurants and fast-food establishments.

Traditionally in Britain and most other western cultures the daily food intake is mainly confined to three specific meal periods: early morning, mid day and early evening. Although the relative quantities of food consumed at each of these meal periods may vary, there is a general adherence to the times. This allows intakes to be controlled in manageable amounts and the nutritional requirements to receive contributions throughout the day.

These habits help enormously in planning the meals. The cardinal rule for athletes, whether eating at home or eating out, is to avoid foods contributing large amounts of fat and to concentrate on those rich in starches. Inevitably, there will be occasions when it is impossible to follow this rule but the advantage of having three meals a day is the possibility of compensating in the meals either before or after the transgression. For example, if you know that it will be difficult to obtain the right foods for the mid day meal, then the breakfast and evening meals should contain a higher proportion of cereal products, fruit and vegetables. In this way the average intake over the day can be brought closer to the target.

Breakfast

The traditional British family breakfast has diminished in recent years and in many households it has virtually disappeared. Breakfast should be an important meal, particularly for those involved in strenuous exercise. Research has shown that people who do not have breakfast can have significantly slower reactions and poorer grip strength by late morning than those who have had an early-morning meal. This appears to be due mainly to their lower blood sugar levels.

As breakfast is the meal most likely to be eaten at home it is often one which can be the most easily controlled.

The wide variety of breakfast cereals on the market gives a good opportunity for complex carbohydrate intake and these should form the basis of the meal. Toast, particularly that made from wholewheat flour, should be another important component.

As the other two main meals of the day traditionally tend to have relatively high fat levels, breakfast should contain the highest possible starch and total carbohydrate content. A typical breakfast could therefore be

200 ml (7 oz) fresh orange juice
35 g (1¼ oz) corn flakes
84 g (3 oz) milk
15 g (½ oz) dried raisins or sultanas
2 slices (62 g) wholemeal toast
7 g (¼ oz) margarine
14 g (½ oz) marmalade
tea or coffee with milk and sugar

total calories	580
carbohydrate	74 per cent (115 g)
fat	17 per cent (11 g)
protein	9 per cent (13 g)
fibre	10 g

The fat content of this meal can be further reduced by using low-fat or skimmed milk. Corn flakes are particularly high in starches and other complex carbohydrates. Other cereals with similar high levels are Rice Krispies (Kellogg's), Grapenuts (General Foods), Ready Brek (Lyons), Puffed Wheat (Quaker), Shredded Wheat (Nabisco), Special K (Kellogg's) and Weetabix.

Muesli tends to have a much lower starch content and higher sugar content, and All Bran (Kellogg's), although having a very high fibre content, also contains about twice the sugar and a third of the starch of corn flakes.

Toast or bread is high in starch, and wholemeal bread contributes useful levels of fibre.

Snacks

To take in the high calorie levels required to sustain normal activity and training, most athletes consume snacks or mini meals between main meals. The pattern of snack consumption is usually fitted around their training habits.

Snacks are also an ideal way to build up the complex carbohydrate intake. A simple snack could be a jam or honey sandwich made with bread or bread rolls. Cream crackers and crispbreads (not starch-reduced) also have high levels of starch and relatively low amounts of sugar. Sweet biscuits and chocolate biscuits contain more sugar.

Cereal and fruit bars (granola bars) make good snacks and usually contain less fat than chocolate-covered bars.

Fruits, both fresh and dried, make good snacks but remember that the carbohydrate content of fruits is made up largely from sugars. Fruits also contribute to the fibre intake. Some vegetables such as celery or raw carrots can make very acceptable snacks especially if eaten with crispbread or savoury biscuits.

If a more substantial snack or light meal is required, this example gives almost exactly the right proportions of energy nutrients:

168 g (6 oz) baked beans in tomato sauce
2 slices (62 g) wholemeal toast
7 g (¼ oz) margarine

total calories	325
carbohydrate	61.5 per cent (53 g)
fat	21 per cent (7.6 g)
protein	17.5 per cent (14 g)
fibre	17 g

This meal is high in fibre which is also advantageous. If 168 g (6 oz) of canned spaghetti in tomato sauce is substituted for the baked beans, the percentage of carbohydrate increases at the expense of protein, and the fibre content is reduced to about 5.5 g per serving. Spaghetti on toast still makes a very acceptable snack meal.

Large baked potatoes with savoury toppings or stuffings also make good mini meals if low-fat stuffings or toppings are used. Ingredients to use for the stuffings include white chicken meat (breast), white fish (cod, haddock, halibut), sweetcorn, baked beans, cooked kidney beans, celery, tomatoes, peppers and mushrooms. These can be mixed with white sauces, pickles or chutneys. Salad creams, mayonnaise or oil-based dressings should be avoided or kept to a minimum. Cottage cheese is a good base for a topping as it is low in fat and high in protein.

Main meals

The selection of suitable main meals will probably cause the greatest problems, as most meals – and particularly those sold in fast-food establishments like fish-and-chip shops – are too high in fat.

If high-carbohydrate breakfasts and snacks have been built into the diet they will help compensate for the extra fat in the main meals. In planning meals the following points should be borne in mind:

reduce the amount of red meat such as beef and lamb and concentrate on white fish and poultry

ensure that a large part of the main course is made up of starch-based serving; this can be boiled or baked potatoes (not roast or chipped), rice or pasta

select a good variety of vegetables and include both dark green (spinach, brocolli) and orange (carrots, pumpkin) vegetables

try and include legumes (peas, beans and lentils) as these are good sources of vegetable protein

desserts should consist of fresh fruit or fruit dishes

if using cheese for cooking or dessert avoid the high-fat cheeses such as Cheddar, Stilton or cream cheese and go for those with lower fat such as Edam, Parmesan and Camembert.

Starters

Most soups are acceptable although the broths made from meat stock, and cream of chicken soups, tend to have a higher fat content than vegetable soups.

Salads are also recommended but watch out for the dressings. A cottage cheese salad is ideal but avoid avocado pears, either on their own or as part of a salad, because of their high fat content.

Main course

For people who prefer the traditional 'meat and two veg' main course the above guidelines are important. As we mentioned, the preferred meat sources are poultry (with the exception of duck), game birds, and fish. These are all good sources of protein with far less fat per serving than beef, pork or lamb. If red meat is on the menu select portions with the least fat, and if possible arrange for as much visible fat as possible to be removed before cooking.

One of the accompaniments to the main course should be a starch-based serving. Traditionally in the United Kingdom this consists of potatoes and they should be either boiled or baked and not roasted or chipped. Rice and pasta make very suitable alternatives to potatoes and can provide variety. Wholewheat pasta, which has now become more commonly available, can contribute to the fibre intake.

Select vegetables to complement the meal. Where possible choose one from the orange/dark green group which are rich in carotenoids. Vegetables particularly high in beta-carotene are broccoli tops, carrots, spinach, pumpkin, spring greens and yellow sweet potatoes. Salad vegetables (eaten uncooked) containing useful quantities of beta-carotene include endive, parsley, watercress and green lettuce. Spinach is a good vegetable to include in a meal because, in addition to the vitamins, it has a relatively high mineral content, particularly the important minerals iron and calcium.

Sweetcorn is a vegetable which is high in starch; in fact on average it has a higher starch content than potato. A serving of sweetcorn can either be used as an alternative to potatoes or as an additional vegetable. As the latter it is a good way of increasing the total carbohydrate level in the meal.

Peas, butter beans, haricot beans, kidney beans and lentils all contain useful quantities of vegetable protein in addition to starch.

All vegetables, particularly green-leafed ones, should be cooked in as little water as possible for the minimum time. To retain as much vitamin and mineral content as possible eat vegetables immediately after cooking.

Salads are particularly rich in vitamins and minerals, but very few traditional salad vegetables contain useful amounts of the energy nutrients as most of them have water contents of between 90 and 95 per cent.

Alternatives to the 'meat and two veg' meals are rice and pasta dishes. Risottos can be prepared with chicken meat (see recipe in appendix 3), and most recipe books give ideas for spaghetti, macaroni and other pasta dishes. It is also worth exploring pasta recipes for vegetarians.

The next example shows the importance of looking for hidden fat in the British diet. The main course is a high-carbohydrate, high-protein, low-fat meal. The course itself is quite substantial in volume and weight (510 g or 1 lb 2 oz), but only contributes 400 calories.

168 g (6 oz) white fish steamed or grilled (cod, haddock or plaice)
112 g (4 oz) boiled potatoes
112 g (4 oz) sweetcorn
56 g (2 oz) spinach

total calories	400
carbohydrate	45 per cent (48 g)
fat	11.5 per cent (5.2 g)
protein	43.5 per cent (44 g)

The reason for this is that white fish (eg cod) contains less than 1.5 per cent fat. If 168 g (6 oz) of grilled rump steak, which has 12 per cent fat, is substituted for the fish the energy content of the meal increases by 54 per cent to 615 calories. This means that the athlete who is assiduously trying to maintain a high-carbohydrate, low-fat regime has to accept that either each meal will be larger in volume than normal or that more snacks are required between meals to satisfy the higher-than-average caloric requirements.

Desserts

Recommended hot desserts are those based on cereals, eg rice, semolina and tapioca milk puddings. Apple crumble made to a low-fat recipe (appendix 3) is a pleasant high-carbohydrate dessert and if wholemeal flour is used in its preparation it will also contribute a useful amount of fibre. Stewed fruit and custard is another good option.

Most other hot puddings such as sponge pudding, suet pudding and pancakes tend to be high in fat.

Consider fruit, either on its own or in the form of a fruit salad, as one of the ideal cold desserts. Jellies are high in carbohydrates in the form of sugar, as are meringues. Ice cream usually contains beteen 35 and 40 per cent fat, and cheesecakes can have fat contents as high as 70 per cent when made with cream cheese.

Cheeses, being in the dairy products group, are generally good sources of calcium. Unfortunately most cheeses also have a high fat content. Parmesan cheese has one of the highest calcium contents with a 28 g (1 oz) portion contributing over two-thirds of the British adult RDA for calcium. The Edam and Cheddar varieties will give about 40 per cent of the RDA per 28 g. Cottage and cream cheeses normally contain very low levels of calcium. Low-fat yoghurts can make a pleasant ending to a meal. In most commercially prepared yoghurts the carbohydrate content comes almost entirely from sugar.

15 Theory into practice (iii): a case study

A good example of the way the diet can be modified to enhance athletic performance is demonstrated by the work of the Shaklee Corporation nutritionists and dietitians with the American Ski Team.

The United States Ski Team travelled widely within the USA and internationally to take part in events, and the skiers had to eat whatever was available in hotels and camps. During some foreign competitions they found that the diet was totally alien to their culture.

In 1980 the team's doctors decided that the skiers' nutritional intake could be considerably improved and they consulted Shaklee Corporation, a nutritional products manufacturer, who had been conducting research into sports nutrition.

A team of nutritionists and dietitians was assigned by the corporation to work with the skiers, and they were helped by members of the Stanford University Heart Disease Prevention Programme.

The first year was spent collecting information on the athletes' diet, particularly the calorie expenditure and nutritional intakes. Most of this data was obtained from comprehensive three-day food diaries recorded at four different times of the year. One diary period was during a training camp, one was kept during an American competition, one during a European competition and one when the skiers were at home.

Analysis of this data showed that the calorie expenditure of the male skiers during training was about 5000 calories while the females consumed approximately 3500 calories.

The diet was found to be very high in fat and low in carbohydrates when compared to the recommended amounts for athletes (fig 20). Although the skiers consumed a variety of foods, the ratios of the energy nutrients were more typical of the American average which is considered to be too high in fat. Interestingly, the values obtained for both male and female skiers at the training camps showed a higher fat and lower carbohydrate intake than for the periods when the athletes were choosing their own menus. Protein consumption worked out to about 2 g of protein per kg of body weight. Cholesterol intake was found to be high, particularly for the male skiers.

Studies on the iron stores of the female Nordic skiers were carried out at Florida State University. Data was collected over a period of twelve months and it showed that the iron stores of those athletes who travelled from competition to competition fluctuated, especially where there were large changes in altitude. In addition there was a statistically significant decrease in the women's iron stores during long competition periods. Whether this was due to dietary influences or the condition known as 'sports anaemia' is not clear.

A definite effect due to altitude was found in the blood haemoglobin and haematocrit values during the skiers' altitude training.

During one part of the study it was observed that more that 50 per cent of the women skiers should be classified as prelatent iron deficient.

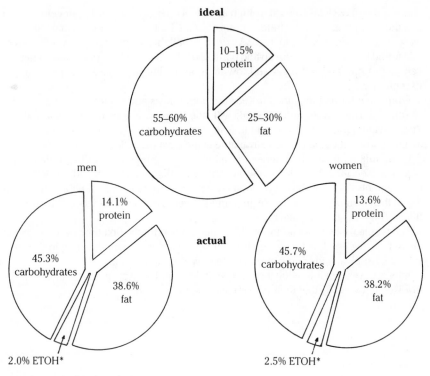

ideal

10–15% protein

55–60% carbohydrates

25–30% fat

men

14.1% protein

45.3% carbohydrates

38.6% fat

actual

women

13.6% protein

45.7% carbohydrates

38.2% fat

2.0% ETOH*

2.5% ETOH*

*alcohol and related products

Fig 20   *Calorie distribution in skiers*

Investigations also showed that the skiers who were provided with a multivitamin-multimineral supplement contributing 18 mg (100 per cent US RDA) per day maintained their iron stores at a higher level than the control group, although they also showed fluctuations at the higher altitudes.

The diaries indicated that calcium intake for the male skiers was well above the recommended daily amount of 800 mg, but approximately 20 per cent of women in one recording session and approximately 40 per cent at another session consumed less than 800 mg.

As a result of information gathered from the diaries, the nutritionists at Shaklee instituted a programme of lectures and literature to encourage better nutritional awareness amongst the skiers and their coaches. The impact of this educational programme was such that there was evidence that the athletes had already begun to make changes to their diets before all the monitoring was completed.

The target was to optimise the Ski Team's diet for the Winter Olympics in 1984, and in preparation for this a nutritionist attended the World Cup events at Sarajevo in February 1983 to evaluate the US team's nutritional intake. The skiers were lodged in a hotel and were being served typical Yugoslavian food. An evaluation of this diet showed it to have a fat content as high as 45 to 47 per cent, about 17 per cent protein and the balance as carbohydrate. A number of the fruits and vegetables that the skiers were accustomed to eating in the USA were not available. During their travels the skiers had found that the mid European and particularly the Eastern Bloc diets were generally very high in fat and red meat and low in good-quality vegetables. Sarajevo was no exception.

From the information gained in 1983 the nutritionists and doctors working with the Nordic Ski Team were able to work with the Olympic medical specialist and the Yugoslavian Agriculture Trade and Industry Department in Sarajevo to obtain a list of all the foods that could be made available at the Olympic Village.

Using this information, a series of guidelines were prepared for the athletes and coaches. The guidelines took into account the different calorie and carbohydrate requirements and were based on foods which were known to be available on a given day at the Olympic Village. These guidelines covered not only solid foods but also the fluid requirements of the skiers.

The whole project was undoubtedly a success and for the first time ever the US Ski Team took five medals including Bill Johnson's gold for downhill skiing in the 1984 Winter Olympics, and is now number one in World Alpine Skiing.

After four years of following the recommended nutritional programme, all the skiers involved felt strongly that their performance had improved.

Appendix 1 The role and sources of vitami[ns] in food

Vitamin	Primary needs in the body	Good food sources	Approximate daily requirement
Vitamin A	Essential for optimum growth and successful reproduction. Important role in vision, especially night vision. Involved in maintaining epithelial cells and mucous membranes.	Liver oils of cod and tuna fish, mammalian liver, egg yolk, milk, green, yellow and orange vegetables	750 μg*
Vitamin B_1 (thiamin)	Essential for key reactions in energy production, particularly in breakdown of carbohydrates. Contributes to the health of the nervous system. Required to maintain healthy heart muscle and is also involved in the functioning of the digestive system.	Cereals (whole grain), yeast, potatoes, vegetables, egg yolk, milk, liver and kidney	0.4 mg per 1000 kcal energy intake*
Vitamin B_2 (riboflavin)	Vital for the metabolism of carbohydrates, amino acids and fats.	Yeast, milk, eggs, liver, kidney, cheese and vegetables	1.6 mg*
Vitamin B_6	Critical for protein and amino acid metabolism. Responsible for synthesis of certain proteins and formation of vital hormones. Important in red blood cell regeneration.	Liver, kidney, cod liver and roe, egg yolk, milk, yeast, cereals	2.0 mg† (no United Kingdom RDA)

Vitamin	Primary needs in the body	Good food sources	Approximate daily requirement
Vitamin B_{12}	Essential in cell division and critical to all cells especially bone marrow and red blood cells, the nervous system and gastrointestinal tract. It works with pantothenic acid in the formation of certain amino acids. It is also required for the synthesis of choline.	Liver, kidney, egg yolk	2 μg*
Biotin	Plays a central role in the synthesis of fatty acids and other compounds in the body. Also appears to be involved in the metabolism of protein and carbohydrates as well as fat.	Liver, yeast, whole grains, mushrooms, milk, some vegetables	0.3 mg† (no United Kingdom RDA)
Vitamin C (ascorbic acid)	Critical to the formation of the protein collagen which binds cells together. Helps maintain healthy gum tissue and teeth. Aids in effective wound healing. Vital in the formation of adrenal hormones and to tryptophan metabolism. Serves as an anti-oxidant and is an aid in iron absorption.	Oranges, grapefruit, blackcurrants, tomatoes, potatoes, and green leafy vegetables	30 mg* (60 mg)†
Vitamin D	Necessary for correct growth and mineralisation of teeth and bones. Helps regulate utilisation and absorption of calcium and phosphorus.	Egg yolk, milk, butter, fish-liver oils (vitamin D can be manufactured by the human body during exposure to sunlight)	10 μg (during winter or during periods of inadequate exposure to sunlight)
Vitamin E	Protects tissues, cell membranes and vitamin A from harmful oxidation processes. Protects red blood cells from rupturing.	Cereal germs, vegetable oils, leafy vegetables, some nuts	12–15 IU† (no United Kingdom RDA)

Vitamin	Primary needs in the body	Good food sources	Approximate daily requirement
Folic acid	Essential in cell division and reproduction. Important for normal growth, especially red blood cells. Responsible for the synthesis of certain amino acids. Works closely with vitamins C, B_6 and B_{12}.	Liver, kidney, wheat germ, milk, cheese, some dark leaf vegetables, mushrooms, shellfish	300 µg*
Vitamin K	Regulates blood coagulation.	Green vegetables, potatoes, tomatoes, strawberries and some liver oils (can be synthesised in human gut by intestinal flora)	About 50 per cent of requirement is manufactured in human intestine. Dietary requirements are probably about 0.5 mg.
Niacin	Forms the active portion of the co-enzymes that release energy from carbohydrates, fats and protein. Also required for synthesis of fatty acids and thus lipids, hormones, and cell membranes required by the body.	Liver and meat of hoofed animals, yeast	18 mg*
Pantothenic acid	Essential for the metabolism of carbo-hydrates, fats and protein including release of energy. Part of a co-enzyme in the formation of fatty acids, cholesterol and many hormones. Responsible for the formation of the neurotransmitter acetyl choline.	Organ meats, egg yolk, yeast, cereals and some green vegetables	10 mg† (no United Kingdom RDA)

* Based on United Kingdom recommended daily amounts.
† Based on United States of America recommended daily amounts.

Appendix 2   Food composition tables

These tables give the composition of some common foods in terms of the three categories of energy nutrients, carbohydrate, fat and protein. The data is based on Paul A A and Southgate D A T (1978) *McCance and Widdowson's 'The composition of foods'* (4th edn), HMSO, London.

The idea of these tables is to provide an indication of the types of food which are relatively high in each of the nutrients. The first table comprises those foods which are good sources of carbohydrates, particularly complex carbohydrates. The second table lists foods which tend to be very high in fat; these foods should be kept to a minimum or excluded from the diet. The third table gives a number of foods which are particularly high in protein.

The symbols on the right of the tables indicate whether the carbohydrate content is high in starches (as opposed to sugar), whether the food is a good source of dietary fibre, and a warning if the food contains a large proportion of fat.

Key

▲   food is a good source of starch and complex carbohydrates
●   food is a good source of dietary fibre
✕   food has a very high fat content

High carbohydrate

Food	Protein	Fat	Carbohydrate		
		g/100 g food			
Flour and cereals					
custard powder (cornflour)	0.6	0.7	92.0	▲	
wholemeal flour	13.2	2.0	65.8	▲	●
brown flour	12.8	2.0	68.8	▲	
white flour (plain)	9.8	1.2	80.1	▲	
macaroni (raw, dry)	13.7	2.0	79.2	▲	
oatmeal (raw, dry)	12.4	8.7	72.8	▲	
rice (raw, dry)	6.5	1.0	86.8	▲	
semolina (raw, dry)	10.7	1.8	77.5	▲	
spaghetti (raw, dry)	13.6	1.0	84.0	▲	
tapioca (raw, dry)	0.4	0.1	95.0	▲	
Bread					
bread, wholemeal	8.8	2.7	41.8	▲	●
bread, brown	8.9	2.2	44.7	▲	
bread, Hovis	9.7	2.2	45.1	▲	
bread, white	7.8	1.7	49.7	▲	
bread, white, toasted	9.6	1.7	64.9	▲	
Breakfast cereals					
corn flakes	8.6	1.6	85.1	▲	●
All-Bran	15.1	5.7	43.0		●
grapenuts	10.8	3.0	75.9	▲	
muesli	12.9	7.5	66.2		
Ready Brek	12.4	8.7	69.9	▲	
Shredded Wheat	10.6	3.0	67.9	▲	●
Weetabix	11.4	3.4	70.3	▲	●

Food	Protein	g/100 g food Fat	Carbohydrate		
Biscuits					
cream crackers	9.5	16.3	68.3	▲	
crispbread, rye	9.4	2.1	70.6	▲ ●	
digestive	9.8	20.5	66.0		✕
shortbread	6.2	26.0	65.5		✕
water biscuits	10.8	12.5	75.8	▲	
Cakes					
gingerbread	6.1	12.6	62.7		
sponge (without fat)	10.0	6.7	53.6		
currant buns	7.4	7.6	54.5		
Vegetables					
butter beans (raw)	19.1	1.1	49.8	▲ ●	
haricot beans (raw)	21.4	1.6	45.5	▲ ●	
lentils (raw)	23.8	1.0	53.2	▲ ●	
potatoes, boiled	1.4	0.1	19.7	▲	
potatoes, baked with skins	2.1	0.1	20.3	▲	
potatoes, instant powder	9.1	0.8	73.2	▲	
potato crisps	6.3	35.9	49.3	▲	✕
sweetcorn, boiled	4.1	2.3	22.8	▲	
sweet potatoes, boiled	1.1	0.6	20.1		
yam, boiled	1.6	0.1	29.8	▲	

Food	Protein	g/100 g food Fat	Carbohydrate
Fruits			
apricots (raw, dried)	4.8	trace	43.4
currants (dried)	1.7	trace	63.1
dates (dried)	2.0	trace	63.9
peaches (raw, dried)	3.4	trace	53.0
raisins (dried)	1.1	trace	64.4
sultanas (dried)	1.8	trace	64.7
Sugar			
white	trace	0	99.9
Demerara	0.5	0	99.3
golden syrup	0.3	0	79.0
black treacle	1.2	0	67.2

High fat

Food	Protein	g/100 g food Fat	Carbohydrate		
Bread					
bread, white, fried	7.6	37.2	51.3	▲	✕
Biscuits					
chocolate, full-coated	5.7	27.6	67.4		✕
sandwich	5.0	25.9	69.2		✕
shortbread	6.2	26.0	65.5		✕
wafers, filled	4.7	29.9	66.0		✕
Cakes					
sponge cake, with fat	6.4	26.5	53.2		✕

Food	Protein	g/100 g food Fat	Carbohydrate	
Pastries				
pastry, flaky	5.8	40.5	47.4	✕
pastry, shortcrust	6.9	32.2	55.8	✕
Puddings				
cheesecake	4.2	34.9	24.0	✕
Dairy products				
butter, salted	0.4	82.0	trace	✕
cream, double	1.5	48.2	2.0	✕
cream, whipping	1.9	35.0	2.5	✕
cheese, Cheddar type	26.0	33.5	trace	✕
cheese, Danish blue	23.0	29.2	trace	✕
cheese, Parmesan	35.1	29.7	trace	✕
cheese, Stilton	25.6	40.0	trace	✕
cheese, cream	3.1	47.4	trace	✕
cheese, processed	21.5	25.0	trace	✕
Eggs				
yolk, raw	16.1	30.5	trace	✕
Fats and oils				
cooking fat	trace	99.3	0	✕
dripping, beef	trace	99.0	0	✕
lard	trace	99.0	0	✕
margarine, all kinds	0.1	81.0	0.1	✕
suet, shredded	trace	86.7	12.1	✕
vegetable oils	trace	99.9	0	✕

Food	Protein	g/100 g food Fat	Carbohydrate	
Meat and meat products				
bacon, cooked	9.3	72.8	0	×
bacon, rashers, fried	24.1	42.3	0	×
bacon, rashers, grilled	24.9	35.1	0	×
beef, roast	22.4	28.8	0	×
lamb breast, roast	19.1	37.1	0	×
lamb chops, grilled	23.5	29.0	0	×
pork chops, grilled	28.5	24.2	0	×
duck, roast	19.6	29.0	0	×
luncheon meat, canned	12.6	26.9	5.5	×
liver sausage	12.9	26.9	4.3	×
Frankfurter sausage	9.5	25.0	3.0	×
salami	19.3	45.2	1.9	×
pork sausage, grilled	13.3	24.6	11.5	×
pork pie, individual	9.8	27.0	24.9	×
sausage roll, flaky pastry	7.2	36.2	33.1	×
Fish				
sardines in oil (plus oil)	19.7	28.3	0	×
sprats, fried	24.9	37.9	0	×
whitebait, fried	19.5	47.5	5.3	×

Food	Protein	g/100 g food		
		Fat	Carbohydrate	
Nuts				
almonds	16.9	53.5	4.3	✕
Brazil nuts	12.0	61.5	4.1	✕
coconut, desiccated	5.6	62.0	6.4	✕
peanuts, roasted, salted	24.3	49.0	8.6	✕
peanut butter, smooth	22.6	53.7	13.1	✕
walnuts	10.6	51.5	5.0	✕

High protein (over 20 per cent dry weight)

Food	Protein	g/100 g food			
		Fat	Carbohydrate		
Cereal and cereal products					
Bemax	26.5	8.1	44.7		
soya flour, full fat	36.8	23.5	23.5	▲	✕
soya flour, low fat	45.3	7.2	28.2	▲	
Milk and milk products					
cows milk, dried, whole	26.3	26.3	39.4		✕
cows milk, dried, skimmed	36.4	1.3	52.8		✕
Cheese					
Camembert type	22.8	23.2	trace		✕
Cheddar type	26.0	33.5	trace		✕
Danish blue type	23.0	29.2	trace		✕
Edam type	24.4	22.9	trace		✕
Parmesan	35.1	29.7	trace		✕
Stilton	25.6	40.0	trace		✕
processed cheese	21.5	25.0	trace		✕

Food	Protein	g/100 g food Fat	Carbohydrate	
Meat and meat products				
bacon, lean, fried	32.8	22.3	0	✕
bacon, lean, grilled	30.5	18.9	0	✕
gammon rashers, grilled	29.5	12.2	0	
gammon joint, boiled	24.7	18.9	0	✕
beef mince, stewed	23.1	15.2	0	✕
rump steak, fried	28.6	14.6	0	
rump steak, grilled	27.3	12.1	0	
sirloin, roast	23.6	21.1	0	✕
stewing steak, stewed	30.9	11.0	0	
lamb chops, grilled	23.5	29.0	0	✕
lamb leg, roast	26.1	17.9	0	✕
lamb shoulder, lean, roast	23.8	11.2	0	
pork chops, grilled	28.5	24.2	0	✕
pork leg, roast	26.9	19.8	0	✕
veal fillet, roast	31.6	11.5	0	
corned beef	26.9	12.1	0	
Poultry and game				
chicken, roast meat only	24.8	5.4	0	
chicken, boiled meat only	29.2	7.3	0	
duck, roast meat only	25.3	9.7	0	
goose, roast meat only	29.3	22.4	0	✕
grouse, roast meat only	31.3	5.3	0	
turkey, roast meat only	28.8	2.7	0	
venison, roast	35.0	6.4	0	
rabbit, stewed	27.3	7.7	0	

Food	Protein	g/100 g food	
		Fat	Carbohydrate
Offal			
kidney, lamb, fried	24.6	6.3	0
heart, sheep, roast	26.1	14.7	0
calf liver, fried	26.9	13.2	7.3
lamb liver, fried	22.9	14.0	3.9
oxtail, stewed	30.5	13.4	0
Fish and fish products			
cod, grilled	20.8	1.3	0
haddock, steamed	22.8	0.8	0
halibut, steamed	23.8	4.0	0
lemon sole, steamed	20.6	0.9	0
herring, grilled	20.4	13.0	0
kipper, baked	25.5	11.4	0
salmon, steamed	20.1	13.0	0
salmon, canned	20.3	8.2	0
salmon, smoked	25.4	4.5	0
sardines in oil (fish only)	23.7	13.6	0
trout, steamed	23.5	4.5	0
tuna, canned in oil	22.8	22.0	0	✕
crab, boiled	20.1	5.2	0
lobster, boiled	22.1	3.4	0
prawns, boiled	22.6	1.8	0
cod roe, hard, fried	20.9	11.9	3.0
herring roe, fried	21.1	15.8	4.7	✕

Food	Protein	g/100 g food Fat	Carbohydrate	
Vegetables				
haricot beans, raw	21.4	1.6	45.5	
red kidney beans, raw	22.1	1.7	45.0	
lentils, raw	23.8	1.0	53.2	
peas, split dried, raw	21.6	1.3	50.0	
peanuts, fresh	24.3	49.0	8.6	✕
peanut butter, smooth	22.6	53.7	13.1	✕

Adapted from Paul AA and Southgate DAT (1978) *McCance and Widdowson's 'The composition of foods'* (4th edn), HMSO, London.

Appendix 3 Recipes

A good selection of high-starch, low-fat recipes can be found in these books:

The F-plan diet, Audrey Eyton, Penguin Books 1982

Audrey Eyton's even easier F-plan, Audrey Eyton, Allen Lane 1984

The high fibre cookbook, Pamela Westland, Martin Dunitz Publishers 1982

Pasta dishes, Janet Hunt, Thorsons Publishers Ltd 1982

Vegetarian cookbooks are also a good source of recipes. A few examples of high-carbohydrate recipes are given here.

Chicken risotto   serves 2–3

220 g (8 oz) diced white chicken meat

8 g (½ tablespoon) vegetable oil

170 g (6 oz) rice

1 chicken stock cube

450 ml (¾ pint) boiling water

55 g (2 oz) mushrooms

40 g (1½ oz) diced mixed vegetables

Heat oil in a medium-size saucepan and fry meat. Add rice and fry for 1 minute. Dissolve stock cube in boiling water and add to meat and rice. Reduce heat and simmer for about 20 minutes or until liquid has been absorbed.

Meanwhile, cook vegetables and add to rice mixture just before serving.

Per 170 (6 oz) serving

energy	211 kcal
	872 kJ
carbohydrate	28.5 g (51 per cent)
fat	5.0 g (21 per cent)
protein	14.6 g (28 per cent)
dietary fibre	1 g

Macaroni and egg

serves 2

2 large eggs

110 g (4 oz) macaroni (preferably wholewheat)

110 g (4 oz) Mexican-style sweetcorn with peppers

2 tablespoons skimmed milk

salt and pepper

Add the macaroni to a large pan of boiling salted water. Bring back to the boil, reduce heat, cover and simmer for 10–12 minutes. Drain and add to the sweetcorn in a saucepan. Beat the eggs with the milk and add salt and pepper to taste. Add to the macaroni and sweetcorn and heat gently, stirring continuously, until the egg becomes creamy and begins to set. Turn out on to serving dish. Serve at once.

Per 170 g (6 oz) serving

energy	307 kcal
	1302 kJ
carbohydrate	50.5 g (62 per cent)
fat	6.4 g (18 per cent)
protein	17.5 g (20 per cent)
dietary fibre	3 g (5 g if wholewheat)

Bread and butter pudding

serves 4–6

7 slices wholemeal bread (crusts removed)

40 g (1½ oz) polyunsaturated margarine

80 g (3 oz) sultanas

70 g (2½ oz) soft brown sugar

3 large eggs

450 ml (¾ pint) skimmed milk

½ teaspoon vanilla essence

freshly grated nutmeg

Butter bread and cut the slices into quarters. Place a layer of bread buttered side up in a greased 1 litre (2 pint) ovenproof dish and sprinkle with half the sultanas and sugar. Add a second layer of bread and sprinkle on the remainder of the sultanas and sugar. Top with a final layer of bread, buttered side up. Whisk the eggs, milk and vanilla essence together and strain over the bread. Leave to stand in a cool place for 30 minutes. Sprinkle nutmeg over the top and bake at 180 °C (gas mark 4) for 25 to 30 minutes until the top is crisp. Serve hot.

Per 170 g (6 oz) serving

energy	287 kcal
	1185 kJ
carbohydrate	41.5 g (54 per cent)
fat	10.5 g (33 per cent)
protein	9.5 g (13 per cent)
dietary fibre	4 g

Apple crumble   serves 2–4

400 g (14 oz) cooking apples, peeled, cored and sliced

100 g (3½ oz) flour

100 g (3½ oz) sugar

50 g (1¾ oz) margarine

½ level teaspoon cinnamon

Arrange apple slices in a dish and sprinkle with half the sugar. Sieve the flour and cinnamon, add remainder of the sugar and rub in the margarine. Spread over surface of the apples. Bake for 40 minutes at 190 °C (gas mark 5).

Per 170 g (6 oz) serving

energy	354 kcal
	1490 kJ
carbohydrate	63 g (67 per cent)
fat	11.8 g (30 per cent)
protein	3.1 g (3 per cent)
dietary fibre	4.3 g

References

American College of Sports Medicine, *Position statement on prevention of heat injuries during distance running*

Anderson J W (1981) *Diabetes.* Martin Dunitz Ltd, London

Barnes G, Morton A and Wilson A (1984) 'Effect of a new glucose-electrolyte fluid on blood electrolyte levels, gastric emptying and work performance', *Australian J of Sci and Med in Sport,* 16(1), 25–30

Bergstrom J and Huttman E (1969) 'Nutrition and maximal sports performance', *J Appl Physiol,* 26, 170–6

Berry Ottaway P (1984) 'Nutrition for gymnasts', *The Gymnast,* May/June

Bodwell C E (1979) 'Human versus animal assays', *Soy protein and human nutrition.* Academic Press, New York

Briggs G M and Calloway D H (1979) *Bogert's nutrition and physical fitness* (10th edn). W B Saunders Company, Philadelphia

Budd M L (1981) *Low blood sugar.* Thorsons Publ Ltd, Northampton

Bylinsky G (1984) 'Closing in on a cure for diabetes', *Fortune,* 6 Aug, 40–3

Cade R, Spooner G, Schlein E, Pickering M and Dean R (1972) 'Effect of fluid, electrolyte and glucose replacement during exercise on performance, body temperature, rate of sweat loss and compositional changes of extracellular fluid', *J Sports Med,* 12, 150–6

Coyle E F, Costill D L, Fink W J and Hooper D G (1978) 'Gastric emptying rates for selected athletic drinks', *The Research Quart,* 49, 119–25

Coyle E F, Hagberg J M, Hurley B F, Martin W H, Ehsani A A and Holloszy J O (1983) 'Carbohydrate feeding during prolonged continuous exercise can delay fatigue', *J Appl Physiol,* 55 (1), 230–35

Crapo P A (1984) 'Theory vs fact: the glycaemic response to foods', *Nutrition Today,* 19 (2), 6–11

Crapo P A and Olefsky J M (1980) 'Fructose – its characteristics, physiology and metabolism', *Nutrition Today,* 15 (4), 2–7

Crapo P A, Scarlett J A and Koctermann O G (1982) 'Comparison of the metabolic response to fructose and sucrose sweetened foods', *Am J Clin Nutr,* 36, 256

Department of Health and Social Security Committee on Medical Aspects of Food Policy (1984) *Diet and cardiovascular disease.* DHSS Report 28, HMSO, London

References

Department of Health and Social Security (1979) *Recommended daily amounts of food energy and nutrients for groups of people in the United Kingdom.* Report on Health and Social Subjects no. 15, HMSO, London

Distiller L A (1980) *So you have diabetes!.* MTP Press Ltd, Lancaster

Dolger H and Seeman B (1984) *How to live with diabetes.* Penguin Books Ltd, England

Durnin J V G A (1985) 'The energy cost of exercise', *Proc Nutr Soc,* 44 (2), 273–82

Ellsworth N M, Hewitt B F and Haskell W L (1985) 'Nutrient intake of elite male and female Nordic skiers', *Phys and Sports Med,* 13 (2), 82–92

Fennema O (1984) 'The placebo effect of foods', *Food Technology,* Dec, 57–67

Fox E L (1979) *Sports physiology.* Saunders College, Philadelphia

Greenleaf J E (1982) 'The body's need for fluid', *Nutrition and athletic performance* (eds Haskell, Scala and Whittam). Bull Publishing Company, Palo Alto

Goldberg L, Elliot D L, Schutz R W and Kloster F E (1984) 'Changes in lipid and lipoprotein levels after weight training', *J Am Med Assoc,* 252 (4), 504–6

Haskell W, Scala J and Whittam J (1981) *Nutrition and athletic performance.* Proceedings of conference on nutritional determinants in athletic performance, Bull Publishing Co, Palo Alto

Hopkins F G (1912) 'Feeding experiments illustrating the importance of accessory factors in normal dietaries', *J Physiol,* 44, 425–65

Howard H and Segesser B (1975) 'Ascorbic acid and athletic performance', *Ann N Y Acad Sci,* 258, 458–64

Jenkins D J A, Wolever T M S, Jenkins A L, Josse R G and Wong G S (1984) 'The glycaemic response to carbohydrate foods', *Lancet,* 388–91

Jenkins D J A *et al.* (11 authors) (1981) 'Glycaemic index of foods: a physiological basis for carbohydrate exchange', *Am J Clin Nutr,* 34, 362–6

Jette M, Pelletier O, Parker L and Thoden J (1978) 'The nutritional and metabolic effects of a carbohydrate rich diet in a glycogen supercompensation training regimen', *Am J Clin Nutr,* 31, 2140–8

Karlson J and Saltia B (1971) 'Diet, muscle glycogen and endurance performance', *J Appl Physiol,* 31, 203–6

Khosla T and McBroom V C (1985) 'Age, height and weight of female Olympic finalists', *Brit J Sports Med,* 19, 96–100

Kirsch K A and von Ameln H (1981) 'Feeding patterns of endurance athletes', *Eur J Appl Physiol,* 47, 197–208

Konopka P and Obergfell W (1980) *Die Gesunde Ernährung des Sportlers.* C D Verlagsgesellschaft, Stuttgart

Levine L, Evans W J, Cadarette B S, Fisher E C and Bullen B A (1983) 'Fructose and glucose ingestion and muscle glycogen use during submaximal exercise', *J Appl Physiol,* 55 (6), 1767–71

McCann J (1980) 'Glycogen–loading just before event may lead quickly to hypoglycaemia', Sports Report, *Medical Tribune,* 4 June

Maughan R J (1981) 'The physiology of injured skeletal muscle', *Sports fitness and sports injuries* (ed T Reilly). Faber and Faber, London-Boston, 193–8

Maughan R J (1984) 'Diet and nutrition: drink', *Running Magazine,* December, 42–3

Maughan R J (1985) 'Fluid and electrolyte balance in prolonged exercise', *Nutr Bull,* 10 (1), 28–35

Mayer J and Bullen B (1960) 'Nutrition and athletic performance', *Physiol Rev,* 40, 369–97

Muckle D S (1981) *Get fit for soccer.* Pelham Books, London, 67–8

Müller-Wohlfahrt H W, Montag H J and Diebschlag W (1984) *Süsse Pille Sport.* Verlag Medical Concept, Munich

National Advisory Committee on Nutritional Education (1983) *Proposals for nutritional guidelines for health education in Britain.* Health Education Council, London

National Dairy Council (1982) *Report on survey of children's eating habits,* London

National Research Council (USA) (1980) *Food and Nutrition Board recommended dietary allowances* (9th edn). Nat Acad Sci, Washington DC

Oakley W G, Pyke D A and Taylor K W (1978) *Diabetes and its management* (3rd edn). Blackwell Scientific Publ, Oxford

Paffenbarger R S, Hyde R T, Wing A L and Steinmatz C H (1984) 'A natural history of athleticism and cardiovascular health', *J Am Med Assoc,* 252, 491–5

Paul A A and Southgate D A T (1978) *McCance and Widdowson's 'The composition of foods'* (4th edn). HMSO, London

Parry S V (1985) 'Biochemistry and physiology of the muscle cell', *Proc Nutr Soc,* 44 (2), 235–43

Pitts G C, Johnson R E and Consolazio F C (1944) 'Work in the heat as affected by intake of water, salt and glucose', *Am J Physiol,* 142, 253–9

Placido V J and Macaraeg J (1983) 'Influence of carbohydrate electrolyte ingestion on running endurance', *Symposium 'Nutrient utilization during exercise',* Ross Laboratories, Columbus, Ohio

Scala J (1981) 'Supplementation for athletes: a training option', *J US Ski Coaches Assn,* 4 (2), 24–6

References

Seiple R S, Vivian V M, Fox E L and Bartels R L (1983) 'Gastric-emptying characteristics of two glucose polymer-electrolyte solutions', *Med Sci Sports Exerc,* 15 (5), 366–9

Sperryn P N (1983) *Sport and Medicine.* Butterworths, London

Taylor R J (1964) *The chemistry of proteins.* Unilever Educational Booklet – Advanced Series, Unilever Ltd, London

Veller O D (1968) 'Studies on sweat losses of nutrients', *Scan J Clin Lab Invest,* 21, 157–67

Welborne T A (1984) 'Diabetes and macrovascular disease: epidemiology, nutritional and environmental factors', *Human Nutrition: Clinical Nutrition,* 38c, 165–74

Williams C (1985) 'Human metabolic response to exercise', *Nutr Bull,* 10 (1), 20–7

Williams C (1985) 'Nutritional aspects of exercise induced fatigue', *Proc Nutr Soc,* 44 (2), 245–56

Wilmore J H (1982) 'Body composition and athletic performance', *Nutrition and athletic performance* (eds Haskell, Scala and Whittam). Bull Publishing Company, Palo Alto

Wootton S (1985) 'Diet and nutrition: the concentration factor', *Running Magazine,* January, 64–7

Yoshimura H (1970) 'Anaemia during physical training', *Nutrition Rev,* 28, 251–3

Recommended reading

Textbooks on nutrition and physiology

Briggs G M and Calloway D H (1979) *Bogert's nutrition and physical fitness (10th edn)*. W B Saunders Company, Philadelphia

Davidson S, Passmore R, Brock J and Truswell A (1975) *Human nutrition and dietetics*. Churchill Livingstone, London

Mitchell H S, Rynbergen H J, Anderson L and Dribble M V (1976) *Nutrition in health and disease*. Lippincott, Philadelphia

Ministry of Agriculture, Fisheries and Food (1976) *Manual of nutrition*. HMSO, London

McNaught A B and Callander R (1972) *Illustrated physiology*. Churchill Livingstone, London

Vander A J, Sherman J H and Luciano D S (1970) *Human physiology*. McGraw-Hill Book Co, New York

Books on sports nutrition

Darden E (1976) *Nutrition and athletic performance*. The Athletic Press, Pasadena

Katch F I and McArdle W D (1977) *Nutrition, weight control and exercise*. Houghton Mifflin Co, Boston, USA

National Assn for Sport and Physical Education (1984) *Nutrition for sport success*. The Nutrition Foundation (USA)

Williams M H (1983) *Nutrition for fitness and sport*. William C Brown Co, Dubuque, Iowa

Food composition tables

The main reference work on the composition of foods in the United Kingdom is:

Paul A A and Southgate D A T (1978) *McCance and Widdowson's 'The composition of foods'* (4th edn). HMSO, London.

This contains information on almost 1000 foods and ingredients and gives compositional data on over 30 nutrients for each food.

A very abridged version of these tables covering 150 foods can be found in

Ministry of Agriculture, Fisheries and Food (1976) *Manual of nutrition*. HMSO, London.

Glossary

Adipose tissue   Tissue consisting of an aggregation of fat cells containing large globules of fat which provides insulation and can be used as an energy reserve.

ADP   Adenosine diphosphate is a nucleotide consisting of adenine, D-ribose and two phosphate groups and is an important co-enzyme in many biological reactions.

Aerobic respiration   A type of cellular respiration in which organic foodstuffs, usually carbohydrates, are completely oxidised to carbon dioxide and water using free oxygen from the atmosphere.

Alcohol   An organic compound that contains one or more hydroxyl (–OH) groups.

Alimentary tract   The tube in animals into which foodstuffs pass to be broken down (ie digested). Succeeding parts of it deal with ingestion, digestion, absorption, egestion. Food is taken in through the mouth and waste egested through the anus.

Amino acid   An organic acid with a free, acidic carboxyl group (–COOH) and a free basic amino group (NH_2). Large numbers of amino acids combine to form protein molecules. Some essential amino acids must be obtained from the diet because they cannot be synthesised by the body.

Anaemia   A disease in which there is a reduction in the amount of haemoglobin in the blood.

Anaerobic respiration   Tissue respiration in which energy as ATP is produced by breakdown of substances in reactions that do not use oxygen.

Anion   *See* Ion.

Antioxidant   A substance that protects body cells against unwanted reactions with oxygen.

Ascorbic acid   Vitamin C.

ATP   Adenosine triphosphate is a nucleotide consisting of adenine D-ribose and three phosphate groups and is the source of energy for most reactions.

Basal metabolic rate   The metabolic rate of the body at rest, ie the energy required to maintain vital processes such as circulation, respiration etc.

Beta-carotene   A photosynthetic pigment found in some plants which the human body can convert into vitamin A (provitamin A).

B-complex   A group of eight water-soluble vitamins, namely B_1, B_2, B_6, B_{12}, niacin, pantothenic acid, biotin, and folic acid.

Bile   An alkaline liver secretion, stored in the gall bladder, which is passed into the duodenum to aid digestion of fats.

Biotin   One of the B-complex vitamins.

BMR   *See* Basal metabolic rate.

Calorie   The amount of heat required to raise 1 g of water from 15 °C to 16 °C. Used as a measure of the energy value of foods. 1000 calories = 1 kilocalorie.

Carbohydrate   A group of complex compounds consisting of carbon, hydrogen and oxygen conforming to the general formula $C_x(H_2O)y$, eg sugars, starch, and cellulose. One of the main sources of energy in food.

Carbohydrate loading   A technique whereby the glycogen reserves in muscle can be increased over the normal levels.

Catalyst   A substance that increases the rate of a chemical reaction without itself being changed at the end of the reaction.

Cation   *See* Ion.

Cellulose   A complex polysaccharide consisting of long chains of glucose molecules linked together. Normally indigestible by humans.

Cholesterol   An animal steroid found mainly in plasma membranes, bile, blood cells and egg yolk.

Chyme   The soft mass of partially digested food as it leaves the stomach.

Co-enzyme   An organic molecule necessary for the activity of some enzymes.

Collagen   The principal structural protein of connective tissue. The main substance which binds cells and tissues together.

Colon   The first part of the large intestine.

Cyanocobalamin   Vitamin B_{12}.

Defaecation   The act of expelling faeces.

Diabetes   A disease caused by insufficient insulin production.

Dietary fibre   The indigestible portion of plant materials consisting of such components as cellulose, hemicellulose, lignin, pectin, and gums.

Digestion   The breakdown by enzymes of complex foodstuffs into simple molecules that can be absorbed by the body.

Disaccharides   Sugars formed by the combination of two monosaccharides, eg maltose, sucrose, lactose.

Diuretic   A substance that causes increased urine production.

DNA   Deoxyribosenucleic acid. A molecule which contains the body's genetic information.

Double bond   A type of linkage between atoms in which two pairs of electrons are shared equally.

Duodenum   The first part of the small intestine. Leads out of the stomach and receives bile and pancreatic ducts. A region of active digestion.

Eicosapentaenoic acid   A 20 carbon atom chain fatty acid with five double bonds.

Electrolytes   Dissolved salts or ions in body fluids which carry electrostatic charges, eg Na^+, Cl^-.

Emulsifier   A substance that reacts in such a way as to enable one liquid to be suspended as fine droplets in another.

Enzymes   Complex protein molecules that act as biological catalysts (*see* Catalyst). Normally enzymes are very specific in the substrates with which they will react. Enzymes are unstable substances easily destroyed or inactivated (eg by heat).

EPA   *See* Eicosapentaenoic acid.

Essential amino acid   An amino acid which cannot be synthesised by the body and must be contained in the diet.

Essential fatty acids   The fatty acids linoleic acid and linolenic acid which cannot be synthesised by the human body and must be taken in from the diet.

Extracellular fluid   The fluids of the body outside the plasma membranes of the body's cells.

Faeces   Residue of undigested food, bile, other secretions and bacteria which is expelled from the anus.

Fat   An organic substance containing fatty acids, glycerol and the elements carbon, hydrogen and oxygen. True fats are solid below 20 °C. Can also be used as an alternative term for adipose tissue (body fat).

Fatty acid   A carboxylic acid.

Folic acid   One of the B-complex vitamins.

Food diary   A record of all food and drink consumed over a set period of time.

Fibre   *See* Dietary fibre.

Galactose   A hexose sugar (monosaccharide).

Gall bladder   A small gland located between the lobes of the liver where bile is stored.

Gastric juices   Secretions from the glands in the stomach wall.

Glucagon   A pancreatic hormone which stimulates the breakdown of glycogen to glucose.

Glucose   A hexose sugar (monosaccharide). Glucose is a major component of disaccharides (eg sucrose) and polysaccharides (eg starch, cellulose, glycogen).

Glycerol   A sugar alcohol.

Glycogen   A soluble polysaccharide (animal starch). It is the form in which carbohydrate is stored in the body and used as an energy reserve.

Haem-iron   Iron of animal origin, eg haemoglobin.

Haemoglobin   An iron-containing blood protein which transports oxygen in the bloodstream.

Hemicellulose   One of a heterogenous group of alkali-soluble polysaccharides including xylans, galactans, mannans. Normally indigestible by humans (*see* Dietary fibre).

Hexose   A monosaccharide with six carbon atoms.

Homeostasis   The maintenance of a stable internal environment within the body.

Hormone   An organic substance produced by endocrine (ductless) glands which help co-ordinate body functions.

Hyperglycaemia   A condition caused by excessive amounts of sugar in the blood.

Hypoglycaemia   A condition caused by low blood sugar levels.

Inorganic substances   Compounds or materials which do not contain carbon atoms.

Insulin   A protein hormone produced by the pancreas which participates in carbohydrate and fat metabolism.

International Unit   A comparative measure of biological activity in related groups of vitamins.

Intestine   Part of the alimentary canal between stomach and anus concerned with digestion and absorption of food and the formation of faeces.

Intracellular fluid   The fluid contained within the plasma membrane of the body's cells.

Ion   A single atom or group of atoms chemically combined that has gained or lost an electron and so has an electric charge. Cations are formed by the loss of an electron(s), eg Na^+; and anions have gained an electron and thus a negative charge, eg Cl^-.

Jejunum The wider, middle part of the small intestine between the duodenum and the ileum. This is the main region for food absorption.

Joule A unit of energy, work or heat. 4.184 Joule = 1 calorie.

Ketosis Excessive amounts of ketones in the body especially associated with *diabetes mellitus*.

Kilocalorie *See* Calorie.

Kilogramme A unit of weight equal to 1000 grammes.

Krebs cycle A cyclic series of reactions catalysed by enzymes whereby pyruvate is oxidised to carbon dioxide, subsequently releasing energy which is stored as ATP.

Lactose A disaccharide composed of a glucose and a galactose molecule chemically combined. Also known as milk sugar.

Lecithin A phospholipid. It contains glycerol, fatty acid, choline and phosphoric acid.

Lignin A complex three-dimensional polymer of variable composition which is a common constituent of plant cell walls and is a component of dietary fibre.

Linoleic acid An unsaturated fatty acid which is required by the body in small amounts. Also wrongly called vitamin F.

Lipid One of a class of compounds which contain long-chain aliphatic hydrocarbons and their derivatives such as fatty acids.

Lymph A colourless fluid obtained from blood by filtration through capillary walls.

Lymphatic system A system of thin-walled tubes that conduct lymph from the tissues into the circulatory system.

Macro mineral Minerals required by the body in relatively large quantities, eg calcium, iron.

Metabolism The sum of all the chemical processes taking place in the body, or parts of it. The processes mainly involve both the breakdown of complex organic molecules to simpler molecules, and the formation of ATP.

Microgramme A unit of weight equivalent to $1/1\,000\,000$ g. Designated mcg or μg.

Micronutrient A nutrient required only in small amounts necessary for the healthy growth of the body, eg vitamins and trace elements.

Milligramme A unit of weight equivalent to $1/1000$ g. Designated mg.

Mineral A naturally occurring substance produced by inorganic processes. It is not of animal or plant origin.

Mol The weight of a substance in grammes, numerically equivalent to its molecular weight. 1 mmol is $1/1000$ of a mol.

Molecule The smallest group of atoms of an element or compound which has a free existence.

Monosaccharides The simplest group of sugars with a general formula $C_nH_{2n}O_n$ where n is usually 3–7.

Niacin One of the B-complex vitamins. Also called nicotinic acid or nicotinamide.

Nutrient A food material which is part of the nutritional requirements of the body.

Octacosanol A 28 carbon atom chain molecule found principally in wheatgerm oil, controversially used by some athletes to increase endurance capacity.

Oesophagus   Part of the alimentary tract, it is a muscular tube that runs from the pharynx to the stomach. It is also known as the gullet.

Osmosis   The passage of solvent molecules across a semipermeable membrane from a less concentrated to a more concentrated solution.

Osteoporosis   A calcium deficiency in adults caused by a failure to absorb calcium as a result of lack of vitamin D or dietary calcium. Bones become brittle.

Oxidation   A process by which oxygen is added to, or hydrogen is removed from, a substance.

PABA   Para-aminobenzoic acid.

Pancreas   A gland which excretes a mixture of enzymes into the duodenum which aid digestion. It also secretes the hormone insulin.

Pantothenic acid   One of the B-complex vitamins.

Pectin   A mixture of acidic polysaccharides found in the cell walls of plants.

Pepsin   A proteolytic enzyme found in gastric juice which breaks down protein molecules into simpler units.

PER   Protein efficiency ratio is a comparative measure of the nutritive quality of a protein.

Peristalsis   Waves of contraction that pass along the smooth muscles of the intestines and similar tubular organs which help to mix the contents of the intestines and passes them from one end to the other.

Pernicious anaemia   A type of anaemia in which abnormal red cells are present in the blood. These cells can only transport very small amounts of oxygen.

pH value   The value on a numerical scale (between 0 and 14) which expresses the acidity or alkalinity of a solution.

Phospholipid   A complex organic phosphorus-containing lipid molecule, eg lecithin.

Photosynthesis   A process in green plants in which complex organic compounds are synthesised from water and carbon dioxide using energy absorbed from sunlight by chlorophyll.

Phytonadione   Vitamin K.

Placebo   A preparation devoid of pharmacological effect given to patients for psychological effect, or control in clinical studies.

Platelet   A very small particle found only in mammalian blood which has an important role in blood clotting.

Polysaccharides   Carbohydrates formed by the combination of a large number (usually the same type) of monosaccharide molecules, eg starch, glycogen, cellulose.

Polyunsaturated   Describes a molecule which has more than one double or triple bond between carbon atoms.

Protein   A complex molecule comprised of many amino acids joined together.

Pylorus   The constriction at the end of the stomach where it leads into the intestines.

Pyridoxine   One of the B-complex vitamins – vitamin B_6.

RDA   Recommended daily amount.

Rectum   The second part of the large intestine where the faeces are stored prior to egestion.

Respiration   The breathing process whereby oxygen is taken from the environment and carbon dioxide is returned to it.

Retinol   Vitamin A.

Riboflavin   Vitamin B_2.

Saliva   A secretion from the salivary glands in the mouth which moistens and lubricates food for swallowing. It also contains some ptyalin, an enzyme, which initiates carbohydrate degradation.

Skeletal muscle   Muscle attached to the bone and under voluntary control.

Starch   A carbohydrate made up from large numbers of glucose units chemically joined together.

Sucrose   Cane sugar, it is a disaccharide composed of a molecule each of glucose and fructose.

Synergism   An action where the total effect of two active components in a mixture is greater than the sum of their individual effects.

Synthesis   The building up of complex molecules from smaller ones.

Thiamin   Vitamin B_1.

Tocopherols   A group of compounds which have varying vitamin E activity.

Trace mineral   A mineral required by the body in very small amounts.

Tryptophan   An essential amino acid.

Urea   An organic compound produced in the liver representing the main nitrogenous waste product of protein breakdown in the body.

Urine   A solution of waste metabolic products produced in the kidney and excreted through the urethra.

Villus (plural: villi)   Any finger-like projection, eg on the wall lining of the small intestine, which greatly increases its surface area.

Vitamin   A complex organic micronutrient required by the body in small amounts.

Index